Barriers of Pap

Smear

REDHWAN AHMED AL-NAGGAR
NOORDIANA BT MAIDEEN

ISBN -10: 1519644396
ISBN-13: 978-1519644398

DEDICATION

This book is dedicated to my family who have been a source of continuous stimulation.

CONTENTS

PREFACE

Globally, cervical cancer is one of the most common cancers in women, with an estimate of 440,000 new cases annually, and 80% of these cases occurring in developing and undeveloped countries. In Malaysia, the population of females in the year 2000 was approximately 10.5 million. Approximately thirty percent of these females are in the reproductive period or older and are at risk of developing cervical cancer. This cancer of the cervix is the second most common cancer among females in Malaysia after breast cancer . There was an average of 2,000-3,000 hospital admission of cervical cancer per year in Malaysia, with the majority of cases presenting at late stages of the disease. In Malaysia, Pap smear screening program commenced in 1969 to ensure early detection of cervical cancer among the target group of women and until the year 2000, only about 850,000 women have undergone Pap smear tests out of the eligible 5.2 million female populations. Nevertheless, only 26% of women in Malaysia had undergone the Pap smear screening, therefore, the purpose of this book is to address the barriers towards Pap smear test.

1 INTRODUCTION

Cervical cancer is malignant neoplasm that forms in tissues of the cervix. It is usually a slow-growing cancer which is asymptomatic but can be found with regular Pap tests. Most cervical cancers are squamous cell carcinomas, arising in the squamous epithelial cells that line the cervix. Adenocarcinoma, arising in glandular epithelial cells is the second most common type. Very rarely, cancer can arise in other types of cells in the cervix.

HPV (human pappilomavirus) is known as the "common cold" of the sexually transmitted infection world. It is very common and affects roughly 80% of all sexually active people, whether they have symptoms or not. The most important risk factor in the development of cervical cancer is infection with a high-risk strain of human papillomavirus. The virus cancer link works by triggering alterations in the cells of the cervix, which can lead to the development of cervical intraepithelial neoplasia, which can lead to cancer. Women who have many sexual partners have a greater risk..

Cervical cancer and its precursor, cervical intraepithelial neoplasia, are more common in women with HIV infection and those infected with HPV subtypes 16, 18, 31, 33, and 35. Most women with cervical intraepithelial neoplasia or cervical cancer are asymptomatic and are found to have the disease by Pap smear. Vaginal bleeding, postcoital bleeding, vaginal discharge, and pelvic pain may occur in women with invasive disease. Biopsy of the cervix confirms the diagnosis of cervical cancer in a woman with an abnormal Pap smear.

Globally, cervical cancer is one of the most common cancers in women, with an estimate of 440,000 new cases annually, and 80% of these cases occurring in developing and undeveloped countries (Masood, 1999). The population of females in Malaysia in the year 2000 was approximately 10.5 million. Approximately thirty percent (30%) of these females are in the reproductive period or older and are at risk of developing cervical cancer. This cancer of the cervix is the second most common cancer among females in Malaysia after breast cancer (Ministry of Health Malaysia, 1999).

The incidence of this cancer is 11.6 per 100,000 populations, with the age standardized rate of 16.2 per 100,000 (Othman, 2006). According to the 2002 report of Malaysia's National Cancer Registry, there was an average of 2,000-3,000 hospital admission of cervical cancer per year in Malaysia, with the majority of cases presenting at late stages of the disease. A year after that, in the 2003 Second Report of the National Cancer Registry of Cancer Incidence in Malaysia showed that cervical cancer constituted 12.9% of total female cancers (National Cancer Registry, 2004). The latest 2005 Social Statistics Bulletin of Malaysia showed that, the death rate due to cervical cancer from 1996 to 2000 ranged from 0.29% to 0.41 % (Social Statistic Bulletin, 2005). According to the National Cancer Registry 2005, a total of 4,057 cases of cervical cancer had been reported from 2003 until 2005.

The age-standardised rate (ASR) of cervical cancer was 16.1 per 100,000 populations. Cervical cancer incidence rate increased with age after 30 years. It has a peak incidence rate at ages 60 - 69 years, and declined thereafter. Chinese women had the highest ASR of 23.2 per 100,000 populations, followed by Indians with ASR of 16.4 per 100,000 populations and Malays with ASR of 8.7 per 100,000 populations (Noor, 2008). Compared to Chinese women in other Asian countries, the incidence of cervical cancer in the Malaysian's Chinese is among the highest.

The Pap Smear Screening Test and its practice in Malaysia.

Pap smear or Papanicolaou's sampling technique, initially developed to study the hormonal status of mice, was a vaginal pool smear, and this is the method originally used in clinical observation on women. It is the screening test that been used to examine any changes in the cervix and facilitates the identification and treatment of precancerous cells before they become symptomatic; which is done by the cytologist or the gynaecologist. The cervical discharge or mucous is taken as a sample by entering the speculum or cervical brush and twist it on the cervical surface. The sample is then smeared on the slide and observed under the microscope.

In Malaysia, Pap smear screening program commenced in 1969 to ensure early detection of cervical cancer among the target group of women and until the year 2000, only about 850,000 women have undergone Pap smear tests out of the eligible 5.2 million female populations (Ministry of Health, 2004). According to the National Cervical Cancer Guidelines 2003 and also Guidebook in Pap smear 2008, all sexually active women age between 20 to 65 years should undergo Pap smear screening annually for two consecutive years and if the Pap smear is normal on both occasions, they can continue the screening test once every three years. Malaysian's Ministry of Health had allocated 3.55 million Malaysian Ringgit in 2003 for the Pap smear screening program. Women who obtain Pap smear test from Public Hospital or other public Health services do not need to pay for the services. (National Health and Morbidity Survey, 1996) Nevertheless, based on the Second National Health & Morbidity Study Report, only 26% of women in Malaysia had undergone the Pap smear screening (Ministry of Health, 2006) and from 1996 until 2005, the total number of Pap smear taken in Malaysia ranged from 350,000 to 400,000 annually and there was no significant increase in the numbers over the years (Noor, 2008).

Factor that influencing the screening.

From these facts, even the disease is seriously affected women but the lower rate of women undergone Pap smear screening for detecting the disease has become a crucial issue to be looked at either for the women, or policy makers themselves in order to overcome this problem. There are inadequate factors known that hinder Malaysian women from taking up screening. Therefore, understanding the factors associated with the underutilisation of cervical cancer screening is important in order to increase overall cancer screening rates. There are several barriers to cancer screening have been identified: these include a lack of awareness of the importance of screening, inadequate access to health care, aversion to the discomforts of screening, fear of finding cancer, age, lack of insurance, socioeconomic factors, low self-esteem, low level of education, never-marriage women and logistic barriers such as having to take time off work for screening (Makinuddin & Ali, 1997; Williams et al., 2002; Bourne et al., 2010). Studies have also revealed that knowledge, attitudes, and beliefs about Pap smear test appeared to be related to actual participation in cervical cancer screening (Urasa & Darj, 2011; Badrinath et al., 2003; Hawkins et al., 2002).

2 BARRIERS OF PAP SMEAR

In a research done by (Al-Naggar et al. 2010) towards 287 female students at a tertiary institution located in Selangor, Malaysia, the prevalence of ever having had a Pap test was 6%. Majority of the participants had adequate knowledge about risk factors of cervical cancer. The highest knowledge about cervical cancer risk factor reported by the respondents was having more than one sex partner (77.5%), whereas the lowest was the relationship between HPV and cervical cancer (51.2%). Age, marital status, ethnicity, monthly family income and faculty were significantly associated with knowledge of cervical cancer screening (p=0.003; p=0.001; p=0.002; p=0.002; p=0.001 & p=0.002; respectively). The most common barriers of cervical cancer screening were the Pap smear test will make them worry (95.8%) whereas the least common barrier reported among participants was no encouragement from the partner.

Attitudes toward cervical cancer and participation in early detection and screening services are well known to be profoundly affected by cultural beliefs and norms. According to (Wong et al. 2008) on their qualitative study conducted with 20 Malaysian women, ages 21-56 years who never had Pap smear; indicates that the respondents generally showed a lack knowledge about cervical screening using Pap smear, and the need for early detection for cervical cancer. Many believed that Pap smear was a diagnostic test for cervical cancer, and since they had no symptoms, they did not go for Pap screening. Other main reason for not doing the screening included; the lack of awareness of Pap smear indications and benefits, perceived low susceptibility to cervical cancer, and embarrassment. Other reasons for not being screened were related to fear of pain, misconceptions about cervical cancer, fatalistic attitude, and undervaluation of own health needs versus those of the family.

According to (Oon et al. 2010) on their qualitative study demonstrated several key findings: Female respondents have better knowledge compared to male. Most of the women perceived that Pap smear screening is beneficial and important, but to proceed with the test is still doubtful. Male respondents were supportive in terms of sending their spouses to the health facilities or give more freedom to their wives to choose and making decision on their own health due to prominent reason that women know best on their own health.

In a study of reproductive health knowledge and cancer screening done by (Chee et al. 2003a) with a total of 486 Malaysian women electronic workers participated showed that the women who ever having a Pap smear was found to be related to being older than 30 years old, being ever married, living with family or relatives, and not staying in hostels. Knowledge on reproductive health was found to be higher for older women, married women, living with family or relatives, not staying in hostels, and ever having had a Pap smear.

In a cross sectional study that was conducted on the knowledge, attitude and practice among midwives and community nurses on cervical cancer in the health service in the state of Kedah in January 1997 (Makinuddin & Ali, 1997) showed that a satisfactory dissemination of information on cervical cancer acquired from radio, tv, newspaper and staff nurses were associated with high level of knowledge on cervical cancer. There were 208 respondents who had Pap smear done. Among reasons for not doing Pap smear were not married (25.8%), embarrassed (25.8%), did not have symptoms (19.4%) and worried about the possible Pap smear result (14.5%). Those who were married, 79.0% of them had Pap smear done.

According to a case control study conducted by (Ab. Karim & Abd. Latip, 1997) showed that there was no significant difference by social-demographic characteristic between cases and controls. Study revealed that 62.2% of cases and 46.2% of control have a high level of knowledge regarding Pap smear. Three aspects of knowledge which contributed significantly to practice were purpose and benefits of the test, places where service is available and risk factors towards cervical cancer ($p < 0.05$). Mean score perception among cases (43.34+5.18) was higher compared to the control group (40.74+6.47), $p < 0.05$. Women's perception towards seriousness of the cervical cancer, perceived benefit of action that is this cancer can be detected earlier before appearance of its signs and symptoms as well as Pap test is not a harmful, discomfort and embarrassing procedure contributed significantly to the practice ($p < 0.05$).

(Chee et al. 2003b) In their cross-sectional survey of women production workers from ten electronics factories showed that the proportion of women who had a Pap smear within the last three years significantly higher among those who were older, married, with young children, on the contraceptive oil or intra-uterine device, had a medical examination within last five years, answered the Pap smear question correctly, and performed BSE monthly.

A lack of knowledge on cervical cancer and the Pap smear test was found among the respondents. Many women did not have a clear understanding of the meaning of an abnormal cervical smear and the need for the early detection of cervical cancer. Many believe the purpose of the purpose of the Pap smear test is to detect existing cervical cancer, leading to the belief that Pap smear screening is not required because the respondents had no symptoms. A quantitative study by (Wong et al. 2009).

The study that examines the determinants of Pap smear Test (PST) screening for cervical cancer among women of different ethnic groups in Malaysia by (Dunn et al. 2009) showed that Indian females are the least likely to have had a PST and also the least likely to know why one is screened. Malay females are less likely than Chinese females to have received a PST and are more likely to report embarrassment as the reason for not being tested. Urban females are less likely than rural females to have been tested and more likely to state lack of time as the reason.

Six hundred eleven (36%) surveys were returned with compliance information. Noncompliance was reported by 33%. Lack of time or inconvenience was cited as the most common reason (93%) for noncompliance, followed by consideration of themselves as low risk for cervical disease (41%) and fear of or embarrassment in seeing a doctor (14%). A survey conducted by (Williams et al. 2002).

According to the study done by (Kahn et al. 1999) stated that the knowledge about Pap smears and pelvic examinations was poor in the 15 interview participants with the mean age was 18.7 years. Most participants believed that their peers receive Pap smears were prevention and early detection or diagnosis, and reported barriers included pain or discomfort, embarrassment, fear of finding a problem, fear of the unknown, denial, poor communication or rapport with the provider, not wanting to look for trouble, lack of knowledge, and peer's advice. Participant-generated strategies for how providers could overcome barriers to Pap smear screening included education ant the development of trusting, consistent relationships with providers.

Socio-demographic factors of Pap smear screening in Taiwan a study done by (Wang & Lin, 1996) shows that substantial evidence exists that regular screening is effective in preventing cervical cancer. However, the existing services are underused by many women in Taiwan. To examine the effects of sociodemographic characteristics on the underuse of Papanicolaou (Pap) smear screening, from September to December 1993 they conducted a questionnaire interview on a sample of 4,400 women aged 20 years and older in Taipei city using multistage sampling with probability proportional to size. Their results indicate that 40% of the women sampled have never had a Pap smear and 86% have not had one in the past year. Age is the strongest factor affecting Pap smear use, particularly for women below age 30 and over the age of 65. In addition, women with lower levels of education, women who are not employed, never-married women who live outside the city tend to underuse Pap smear screening.

A cross sectional survey consisting of a questionnaire of 650 randomly selected women aged 15 to 78 years was performed by (Yu & Rymer, 2003) to gain an insight into women's attitudes to and awareness of smear testing and cervical cancer. Of the respondents, 80.5% had had at least one smear test and 71.5% of these women have regular smears. The majority of the women (66.9%) thought the test 'no problem' and those who found the test 'embarrassing, painful or troublesome' were of a younger age group. Overall, 76.2% perceived the disease to be a common one. 32.6% of the respondents thought the age group 40s to 50s to be most affected by cervical cancer. On the whole, women appeared to be well informed of the link between the number of sexual partners and cervical cancer as well as recognising smoking to be a contributing factor. A substantial proportion (91.7%) of women was of the attitude that cancer can be treated if detected early enough. The perceived barrier such as embarrassment and discomfort played a part in women's decision in returning for a regular smear.

In a study by (Oscarsson et al. 2008) with objective to describe and interpret why women with no cervical smear taken during the previous 5 years choose not to attend a cervical cancer screening (CCS) programme, the following themes were revealed: I do not need to..., I do not want to... and I do not give it priority.... The women had a positive attitude to CCS but as long as they felt healthy, they chose not to attend. A negative body image, low self-esteem, feelings of discomfort when confronted with the gynaecological examination and fear of the results also influenced their non-attendance. The women prioritized more important things in life and reported various degrees of lack of trust in health-care.

(Allahverdipour & Emami. 2008) in their studies of Perceptions of cervical cancer threat, benefits, and barriers of Papanicolaou smear screening programs for women in Iran found that a total of 68.5% reported having undergone at least one Pap test. Women were more likely to participate in Pap smears when they had access to knowledge about cervical cancer and screening programs. Furthermore, the perceived benefit and barrier variables of the Health belief model were two factors related to participation in Pap smear testing.

The relative effects of race/ethnicity and other sociodemographic factors, compared to those of attitudes and beliefs on willingness to have cancer screening, are not well understood. According to (Kressin et al. 2010) based on their study of Self-reported willingness to have cancer screening and the effects of sociodemographic factors among telephone interviews with 1148 adults (22% Hispanic, 31% African American, and 46% white) found that racial/ethnic minority status, age, and lower income were frequently associated with increased willingness to have cancer screening, even after including attitudes and beliefs about screening. Having screening nearby was important for community screening, and anticipation of embarrassment from screening for when there were no cancer symptoms.

Factors influencing cancer screening practices of underserved women. This integrated review was conducted by (Ackerson & Greteback, 2007) to evaluate the factors that inhibit or promote decisions by African American and Hispanic women to obtain cervical cancer screening. They found that cervical cancer screening practices of African American and Hispanic women were influenced by extrinsic motivators including lack of insurance, no usual source of health care, acculturation, and socioeconomic factors. Intrinsic motivators were related to beliefs and perceptions of vulnerability, such as ignoring cervical cancer screening when no symptoms were present; believing that not knowing if one had cervical cancer was better; and thinking that only women who engage in sexual risk-taking behaviours need to obtain Papanicolaou (Pap) smear testing.

(Harlan, et al. 1991) on their interview survey data of Cervical cancer screening: who is not screened and why? found that the results indicates through age 69, Blacks are screened at similar or higher rates than Whites. Hispanics, particularly those speaking only or mostly Spanish, are least likely to have received a Pap smear within the last three years. Of women who had never heard of or never had a Pap smear, nearly 80 percent reportedcontact with a medical practitioner in the past two years, while more than 90 percent reported a contact in the past five years.Overall, the most frequently reported reason for not having a recent Pap smear was procrastinating or not believing it was necessary.

3 ANALYSIS OF CURRENT SITUATION

The convenience method using self-administered questionnaire was conducted among Tengku Ampuan Rahimah Hospital's patients, focusing on the women who visited the Obstetrics and Gynaecology (O&G) Clinics. The questionnaires will be given randomly to the patients that came to the clinics base on inclusion and exclusion criteria.

The study was conducted at the Obstetrics & Gynaecology (O&G) clinics at Tengku Ampuan Rahimah Hospital, Klang and Sg. Buloh Hospital, Selangor. The Tengku Ampuan Rahimah (TAR) General Hospital is a 28-ward Malaysian government medical facility with over 850 inpatient beds patients and 20 clinical disciplines. It has a monthly average of 10,000 and a daily average of 20 elective surgeries.

The Klang TAR Hospital is also a referral hospital for many district hospitals and health clinics ranging from Kuala Langat Kuala Selangor emergency ward. Its Pathology Department conducts over 1,000,000 medical tests helipad in the south up to in the north. It was awarded the MS ISO 9002 Quality System certification in 1998. The hospital has the country's second busiest every year. This hospital also focuses on ambulatory services and is equipped with a for emergency evacuation purposes.

The population for this study was the women who visited the O&G clinics at the hospital. The study involved 142 multiracial patients who come from the different area at Klang Valley. Their participation was voluntary and their feedbacks were anonymous. Ethically, confidentiality was ensured and written consent was obtained.

The samples that were eligible for this study generally must be 18 years and above, specifically only towards female patients and the healthy volunteers that came together with the patients are accepted. The inclusions criteria include the female patients who are more than 18 years and have the ability to speak and clearly understand Malay since the medium of language used in questionnaire were in Malay. On the other hand, the exclusion criteria include women who are under the age of 18, older than 70 years and unable to understand the Malay language.

This study approximately took about two months. It started from September 2011 and ended in November 2011. The questionnaires were distributed around the waiting area in the clinics during clinics hours from 9.00 A.M until 1.00 P.M during weekdays. They were answered anonymously and completed on the spot.

This study begins by getting the approval letter from the Management and Science University in order to ask a permission to conduct this study outside the campus, as a proof that this study is valid and to convince the target sample. After that, the official letter was sent to the Director of HTAR in order to get permission to conduct this study at their place. Afterwards, the director sent the information to the Head of Department of the O&G clinic and after being interviewed and gave a brief explanation about this research, approve were accepted. Each day, the permission from the head of nurse must be gained before starts the distribution. And after that, the consent letter was then given to the participant in order to get their permission to be part of this research.

The sample chosen was done randomly using the convenience method. About 142 respondents were involved. The questionnaires were distributed amongst female patients who visited the Obstetrics and Gynaecology (O&G) clinics (particularly at the waiting area) at the hospitals randomly base on inclusion and exclusion criteria. It was a self-administered questionnaire that is needed to be filled and answers by the participants themselves and was distributed for a month until the targeted number of participant reached.

Ethically, the consent form (refer at Appendix) was given to each respondent as to make sure that the respondent was willing to fill the questionnaire without any constraint. The questionnaires were distributed during their waiting hours without disturbing any of their official matter with the doctor.

The patients were asked if they were willing to complete these questionnaires. All participants were provided with a full explanation on the purpose of the study and how to fill the form. They were asked to answer all the items given and were told that the investigator would be around in order to answer any inquiry regarding the questions. As one returned back those questionnaires, the investigator ensured that everything had been filled in, if not, the participant was asked to fill any missing responses before she left the clinics.

All subjects were surveyed using questionnaires that consist of 33 questions covering the aspects of socio-demographic such as the respondent's age, race, education, occupation, husband's occupation, family monthly income, marital status, age during marriage, number of partner, and menopause status. Also attached together with the questionnaires were questions about the Pap smear test. These include the source of information, the practice and the barriers of Pap smear test. On the last sections, the questions comprised of knowledge and perception towards Pap smear Test. This section was done to explore the deep knowledge about Pap smear test. The questions include the usage of Pap smear, frequency, perceptions and information about this screening test. This part was important as the indicator of the level of knowledge and awareness of the respondents.

Data entry and analyses are undertaken using the Microsoft Excel to be easier presented. Once the entire questionnaires are completed, all the data will be recorded and key in into the computer. The raw data will be calculated by using the Statistical Package for Social Sciences (SPSS) version 16.0 software for window in order to get the results from which will generate a conclusion. Statistical descriptive had been done in order to give the view of frequency and percentage of answers in every question. The obtained results were present in forms of tables and figures. 17

Out of 150 questionnaires distributed, only 142 could be collected.
Out of that, all were answered completely, giving the response rate of
94.67%.

Table 4.1.1: Sociodemographic.

Variable	Value	Frequency	Percent (%)
Age (years)	18-20	14	9.9
	21-30	58	40.8
	31-40	53	37.3
	41-50	15	10.6
	51-60	2	1.4
Race	Malay	88	62.0
	Chinese	13	9.2
	Indian	37	26.1
	Others	4	2.8
Education Level	Never in school	1	0.7
	Primary school	8	5.6
	Secondary middle school	27	19.0
	High school	68	47.9
	Tertiary education	38	26.8
Occupation	Working	60	42.3
	Housewife	69	48.6
	Self-employed	6	4.2
	Not yet working	5	3.5
	Students	2	1.4
Family Monthly Income	Less than RM999	17	12.0
	RM1000-RM2999	74	52.1
	RM3000-RM4999	34	23.9
	RM5000-RM6999	14	9.9
	RM7000-RM8999	2	1.4
	RM9000 and more	1	0.7

Most of the respondents, which is about 58 (40.8%) of them, are aged between 21 to 30 years old and respondents who are 51 to 60 years are the least with about 2(1.4%). However, 53 (37.3%) of respondents, are aged between 31 to 40 years old. This is followed by 15 (10.6%) respondents who are ranged from 41 to 50 years old. About 14 (9.9%) are aged between 18 to 20 years.

Out of 142 respondents, the Malays ethnic group constituted the majority by 88 (62.0%) people. This is followed by the Indians, with 37 (26.1%) and Chinese, 13 (9.2%). The 'others' ethnic group which are about 4 (2.8%) are from Borneo.

From all of these women who responded, the most with about 68 (47.9%) of them were graduated from high school, and 38 (26.8%) were graduated from tertiary education. While the rest, about 27 (19.0%) finished the secondary middle school and 8 (5.6%) were until primary school. And only about 1 (0.7%) of the respondents were never been in school.

Majority of the women, that is 69 (48.6%) are housewife and on the other hand, 60 (42.3%) are working. The remaining of the respondents, who are self-employed, not yet working and students, constitutes about 6 (4.2%), 5 (3.5%), and 2 (1.4%) respectively.

Most of the respondents come from families with a monthly family income ranging from RM1000 to RM2999 with the numbers of respondents of 74 (52.1%) people. This is followed by those families with their income ranged between RM3000 to RM4999, which is 37 (23.9%) of them. The rest, that is ranged from less than RM999 constituted about 17 (12.0%) people, about 14 (9.9%) are between RM5000 to RM6999 and 2 (1.4%) ranged from RM7000 to RM8999. And only 1 (0.7%) of these respondents gained RM9000 and more a month.

Table 4.1.2: The Reproductive Background.

Variable	Value	Frequency	Percent (%)
Marital Status	Single	16	11.3
	Married	124	87.3
	Divorced	1	0.7
	Widowed	1	0.7
Age at first marriage (years)	Not married yet	16	11.3
	14-20	30	21.1
	21-25	60	42.3
	26-30	31	21.8
	31-35	5	3.5
Is your current husband/partner is your first partner?	Not married yet	16	11.3
	Yes	122	85.9
	No	4	2.8
Number of current husband/partner?	Not married yet	16	11.3
	1	122	85.9
	2	4	2.8
Number of pregnancy (including miscarriage)	Not married yet	16	11.3
	Never had pregnancy	17	12.0
	1	24	16.9
	2	25	17.6
	3	26	18.3
	4	14	9.9
	5	9	6.3
	6	8	5.6
	7	2	1.4
	10	1	0.7
Have You had menopause?	Yes	1	0.7
	No	141	99.3
How long have You been menopause?	Not menopause	141	99.3
	6 months	1	0.7
Age at the time of menopause	Not menopause	141	99.3
	49 years	1	0.7

Majority of the respondents are married which account about 87.3%. The single women constitute about 11.3% while the divorced and widowed women are about 0.7% each.

These women get married mostly during 21 to 25 years old which involves the majority of 42.3%. About 21.8% get married between 26 to 30 years old and 21.1% were between 14 to 20years of age. 3.5% get married between 31 to 35 years and 11.3% are still single.

When asked about the status of their current husband/partner, 85.9% of them said he is their first partner and 2.8% said he is theirs second. About 11.3% are still not married.

Among these women, 12% never had pregnancy. With reference to 16.9%, had experienced once or currently being pregnant. 17.6% of the respondents were experienced two, 18.3% had three and 9.9% were having 4 times of pregnancy. Whereas 6.3% of these women experienced five times, 5.6% six times and 1.4% seven times. Out of these, 0.7% was having 10 number of pregnancy. The remaining 11.3% are not married women.

For this section, only 1 (0.7%) of women had menopause which started last 6 months from the day of surveyed. And this woman was in her 49 years old of age at the time of menopause. The residual 99.3% are not menopause yet.

THE KNOWLEDGE:

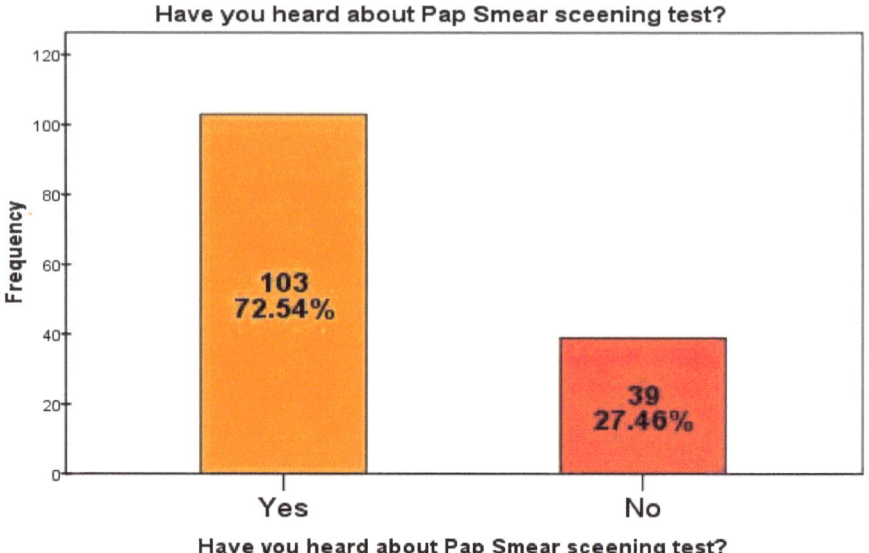

Figure 4.1.1 The Distribution of the women who have heard of PST

Most of the respondents have heard about Pap smear screening test which accounts about 72.54%. In contrast, 27.46% of these women never heard about it before.

Table 4.1.3: The knowledge about Pap Smear Test

Variable	Value	Frequency	Percent (%)
What is the purpose of	Detection of Cervical cancer	105	73.9
PST?	Detection of sexual transmitted disease	3	2.1
	Detection of AIDS/HIV	0	0.0
	Don't know	34	23.9
How often should PST	Once a year	54	38.0
been done?	Once in 1-3 years	26	18.3
	Once in 5 years	2	1.4
	Once in a life time	1	0.7
	Don't know	59	41.5
Can women be forced to	Yes	36	25.4
do the PST?	No	65	45.8
	Don't know	41	28.9

When asked about the purpose of the test, majority of the respondents knows it is for detection of cervical cancer which gives about 73.9% and 2.1% of them said it is for the detection of sexual transmitted disease. However, no one answered is for the detection of AIDS/HIV and 23.9% of these women don't know the purpose of the test.

The next questions were asked about how often should they do the PST and among all, 38% said it should be done once a year, 18% said once in 1 to 3 years, whilst 1.4% said it is done once in 5 years. Regardless, about 0.7% said the PST should be done once in a life time, and the rest about 41.5% don't know how often the test should being done.

These women are also agreed that women cannot be forced to do the PST which gives the 45.8% while still some women said that women can be forced to do the test. Despite, about 28.9% of the women don't know about it.

Table 4.1.4: The opinion about which group of women that should undergo PST

Variable	Value	Frequency	Percent (%)
Married	Yes	114	80.3
	No	28	19.7
Not Married	Yes	39	27.5
	No	103	72.5
Have the family history of cervical cancer	Yes	110	77.5
	No	32	22.5
Had menopause	Yes	38	26.8
	No	104	73.2
Not yet menopause	Yes	46	32.4
	No	96	67.6
Have the symptoms of cervical cancer	Yes	109	76.8
	No	33	23.2
Want to conceive	Yes	36	25.4
	No	106	74.6
Before delivery	Yes	28	19.7
	No	114	80.3
After delivery	Yes	56	39.4
	No	86	60.6

The respondents also being asked their opinion about which group of women should undergo the PST and up to 80.3% agree the married women should do this and 27.5% also agree that even though the women are not married, they should do it too. The highest percentage which is about 77.5% said women who have the family history of cervical cancer and 76.8% of women agree with women who have symptoms of cervical cancer must do it as well. Out of the respondents. 26.8% and 32.4% of them agree women who already had menopause and who is not menopause yet are also must to do the PST, respectively. At the same time, 25.4% of the women agreed that the women who want to conceive can also do it. It is quite interesting to know that about 19.7% and 39.4% of the respondents respectively agreed that women should do the PST before and after delivery. However, there are still a large number of the women who are not agreeing in some aspect of types of women stated above.

Table 4.1.5: The basic knowledge about cause of cervical cancer

Variable	Value	Frequency	Percent (%)
Do you know that cervical cancer is caused by viral infection?	Yes	94	66.2
	No	48	33.8
Do you know that this infection is caused by sexual intercourse?	Yes	70	49.3
	No	72	50.7

There are about majority of the respondents know that cervical cancer is caused by viral infection, generally, which is up to 66% and about 33.8% were not able to acknowledge it. Mean while, 49.3% know that the viral infection is gained from sexual intercourse and 50.7% doesn't know about it.

Table 4.1.6: From which source did you heard about PST

Variable	Value	Frequency	Percent (%)
Doctor/Hospital/Clinic	Yes	82	57.7
	No	60	42.3
Printed Media (Newspaper, magazine, books, flyers, etc)	Yes	62	43.7
	No	80	56.3
Electronic Media (Radio, television, etc)	Yes	45	31.7
	No	97	68.3
Family/Relatives/Friends	Yes	37	26.1
	No	105	73.9
Workplace/Employer	Yes	18	12.7
	No	124	87.3
Internet	Yes	31	21.8
	No	111	78.2
Others	Yes	1	0.7
	No	141	99.3

This table shows various sources of information regarding the Pap smear test. Approximately, 57.7% of the respondents said that they receive the information from the doctor, hospital or clinics. 43.7% of them said that they have read it from the printed media such as newspaper; magazine, books, flyers and etc. 31.7% said they gained it from the family, relatives or friends. In addition, 12.7% respondents get the information from their employer or workplace, 21.8% get it from the internet and others including exhibition or booth constitutes about 0.7%.

THE PRACTICES AND BARRIERS:

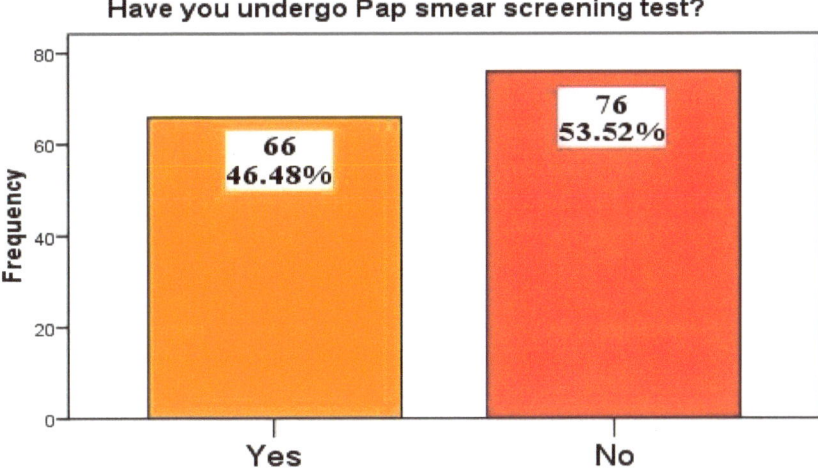

Figure 4.1.2: The distribution of PST practice

The distribution of Pap smear screening test practice is as displayed in figure 4.1.2. As we can see, less than half of the respondents have practice the Pap smear test which is around 46.48%. On the other hand, 53.52% of these women never had Pap smear test before.

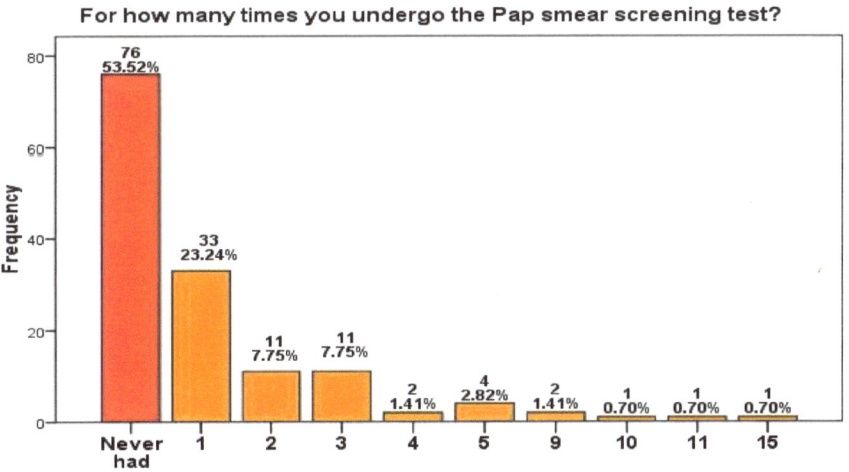

Figure 4.1.3: The distribution of the rate of PST

This figure shows the rate of the Pap smear test being done by these women. Around 23.24% of the respondents had undergo PST once, including their first time, 7.75% did it twice and three times respectively. For the women who did it four times, it is about 1.41%, and five times constitutes about 2.82%. Remarkably, there are women who did it about nine times which give the 1.41% and 0.7% each for 10, 11 and 15 times. Likewise, 53.52% of the respondents never did the test.

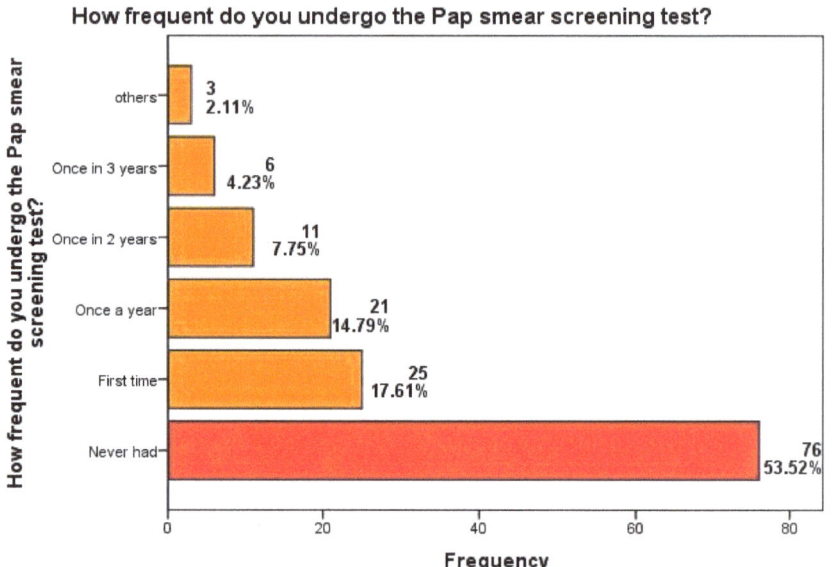

Figure 4.1.4: The distribution of frequency of PST being done

Neglecting the women who never did the PST which took about 53.52%, about 17.61% of the respondents did the PST first time (once). Whereas, 14.79% do it once a year, 7.75% once in two years and 4.23% do it once in three years. Whilst others which take up 2.11% do it only when necessary and twice a year depend on the situation.

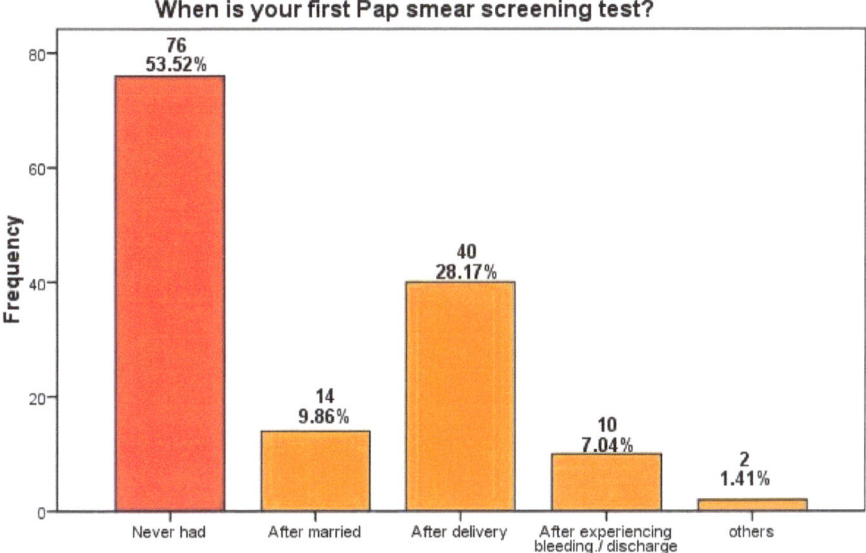

Figure 4.1.5: The distribution of the situation which starts the PST

Figure above shows the situations which lead the PST to be started. As showing above, most of the respondents start doing the PST after delivery which gives the 28.17%. Second most, about 9.86% do it after married, and 7.04% do it after experiencing vaginal bleeding or discharge. The others which is 1.41% of the respondents doing it during pregnancy and after a year on contraceptive pills intake. As mentioned before, 53.52% of the respondent never had PST.

Table 4.1.7: The first and last year of the PST

Variable	Value	Frequency	Percent (%)
In which year you went for PST?	Never doing	76	53.5
	1993	2	1.4
	1996	2	1.4
	1997	3	2.1
	1999	1	0.7
	2000	1	0.7
	2001	5	3.5
	2002	5	3.5
	2003	3	2.1
	2004	4	2.8
	2006	2	1.4
	2007	7	4.9
	2008	5	3.5
	2009	8	5.6
	2010	9	6.3
	2011	9	6.3
When is your last PST?	Never doing	76	53.5
	1997	1	0.7
	1999	2	1.4
	2001	1	0.7
	2002	1	0.7
	2004	6	4.2
	2006	1	0.7
	2007	3	2.1
	2008	4	2.8
	2009	8	5.6
	2010	22	15.5
	2011	17	12.0

The earliest year which the respondents did the PST was in 1993 which is about 1.4% and the latest year they did was on 2011 which is around 12.0%. As we can see the pattern of the distribution, the occurrence of the screening test being done is proportionally increasing by year.

Table 4.1.8: Why did you undergo the PST

Variable	Value	Frequency	Percent (%)
For health purpose	Yes	43	30.3
	No	99	69.7
For detection of cervical cancer	Yes	52	36.6
	No	90	63.4
From doctor's advise	Yes	29	20.4
	No	113	79.6
Family/Relatives/Friends/Employer influence	Yes	6	4.2
	No	136	95.8
There are symptoms of cervical cancer	Yes	4	2.8
	No	138	97.2
Want to conceive	Yes	14	9.9
	No	128	90.1
Examination before pregnant	Yes	8	5.6
	No	134	94.4
Examination after delivery	Yes	17	12.0
	No	125	88.0
Family history of cervical cancer	Yes	3	2.1
	No	139	97.9
Death of the family/relatives/friends caused by cervical cancer	Yes	3	2.1
	No	139	97.9
Never had PST	Yes	76	53.3
	No	66	46.5
Others	Yes	2	1.4
	No	140	98.6

In this section, the question sets to determine the reasons of why the respondents did the PST. Among all, out of 100% in each question; 30.3% of these women did the PST for the health purpose, the highest of 36.6% did for detection of cervical cancer and 20.4% due to doctor's advice. Influence from the family, relatives, friends or employer also contribute about 4.2% and 9.95 of them did it as a reason of wanted to conceive. 5.6% did as part of examination before pregnant and 12% due to examination after delivery. Never the less, 2.1% constitutes each in the reason of had a family history of cervical cancer and death of individuals caused by cervical cancer. These factors influenced them. Others which take up 1.4 % did because of pathological conditions such as appearance of tumour.

Table 4.1.9: Why you do not undergo PST?

Variable	Value	Frequency	(%)
Don't know/ Never heard about PST	Yes	47	33.1
	No	95	66.9
Think it is not important	Yes	11	7.7
	No	131	92.3
Fear	Yes	14	9.9
	No	128	90.1
Embarrassment	Yes	11	7.7
	No	131	92.3
Don't care	Yes	4	2.8
	No	138	97.2
No female doctor	Yes	3	2.1
	No	139	97.9
Expansive	Yes	6	4.2
	No	136	95.8
Don't have time/ busy	Yes	16	11.3
	No	126	88.7
No encouragement from husband/family/friends	Yes	10	7.0
	No	132	93.0
Against your religion/culture/principe	Yes	0	0.0
	No	142	100.0
Distant hospital/clinic	Yes	3	2.1
	No	139	97.9
Painful	Yes	7	4.9
	No	135	95.1
Pap smear makes me worry	Yes	5	3.5
	No	137	96.5
Loss the virginity	Yes	3	2.1
	No	139	97.9
Don't know where to get the PST	Yes	22	15.5
	No	120	84.5
Had done PST before	Yes	66	46.5
	No	76	53.5
Others	Yes	2	1.4
	No	140	98.6

According to the questions, we can clearly determine what factors that prevent these women from undergo the Pap smear screening test. This table shows the reason why they don't do the PST. 33.1% of the women said they don't know or never heard about PST, while 7.7% think it is not important. Similarly, 9.9% of the women are fear and 7.7% feel embarrassed to do the test. Even thought the PST is important, yet 2.8% don't care about the significant of the test. While about 2.1% agreed that there are no female doctor, 4.2% said it is expensive and 11.3% of these women are busy and don't have time. In the same way, due to no encouragement from the husband, family or friends is the reason of why 7.0% of the women don't do the test. Distant hospital or clinic contributed about 2.1%, 4.9% thinks it is painful, 3.5% said the results of the test will make them worry and around 2.1% scared to loss the virginity. Not impressively, 15.5% of these women don't know where to get the PST. Nearly half of the respondents which are 46.5% had done the PST before. Others reason constitutes about 1.4% and among the reason are they did the appointment before but still not being called and one of the women said she is not ready yet.

THE ATTITUDE:

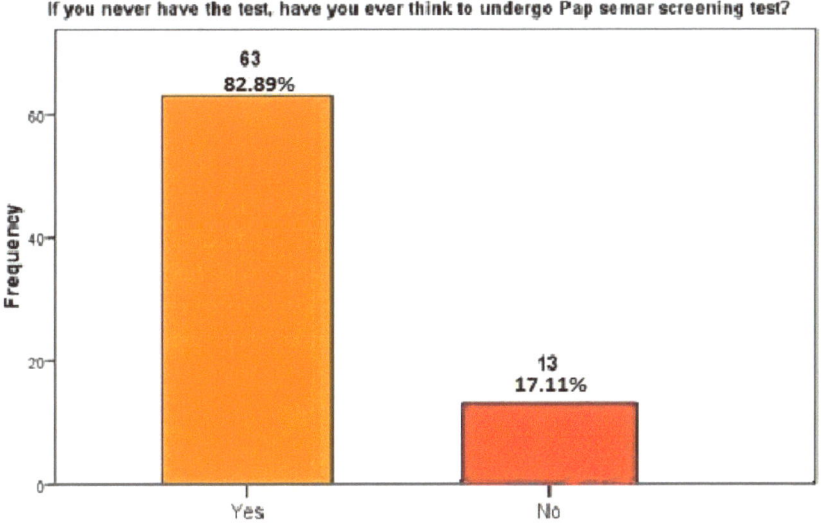

Figure 4.1.6: The intention of obtaining the PST

Table above shows the distribution of the intention to obtain the PST among the respondents. Nearly 44.37% of the women who never do the Pap smear agreed to do the test in the near future and 9.15% said they will not do. While, 46.48% of these women had done the PST.

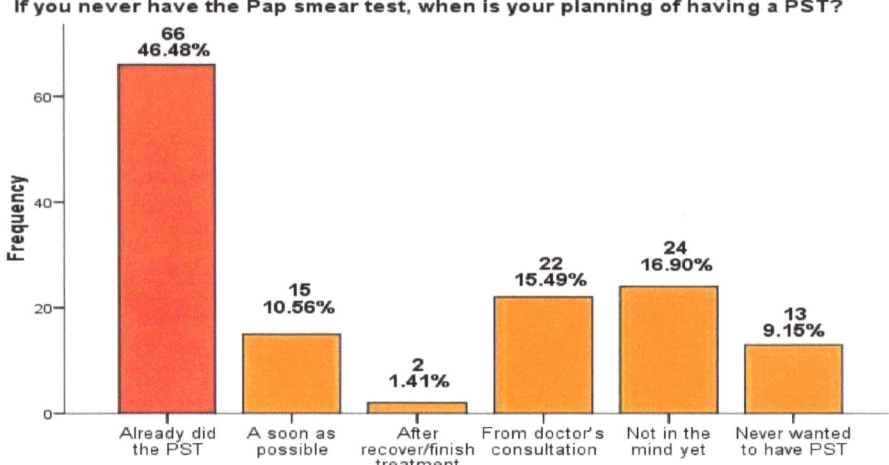

If you never have the Pap smear test, when is your planning of having a PST?

If you never have the Pap smear test, when is your planning of having a PST?

Figure 4.1.7: The distribution of the planning of having a PST

Based on the intention to do the PST, 16.9% of the women not sure exactly when they will do it, while 15.49% will do it after get a doctor's consultation. 10.56% of the respondents said they will do it as soon as possible, whereas 1.41% going to do the PST after recover or finish the treatment. On the other hand, 9.15% of the women never wanted to have it and 46.48% already did the PST before.

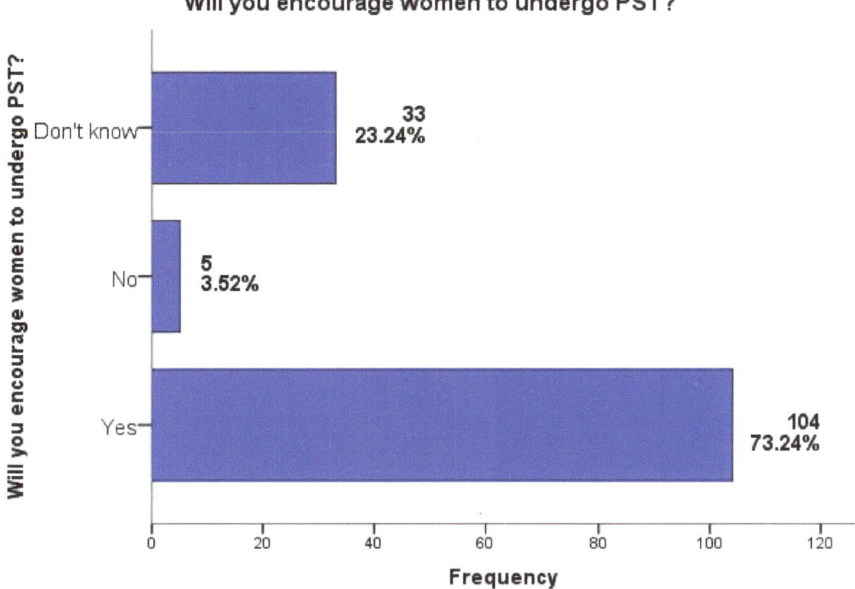

Figure 4.1.8: The distribution of the women who will encourage others to do the PST

The respondents also being asked whether they will encourage other women to do the PST or not and this is how they reacted. Majority of the women said they will encourage other women and 3.52% said they will not. Nonetheless, 23.24% of them placed in don't know state.

Table 4.2.1: The reasons that influenced women to do the PST

Have you undergone PST?	Reasons		Yes	No
Yes				
Count/%				
	For detection of cervical cancer		52 (78.8%)	14 (21.2%)
	For health purpose		43 (65.2%)	23(34.8%)
66	From doctor's advice		29 (43.9%)	37 (56.1%)
100%	Examination after delivery		17 (25.8%)	49 (74.2%)
	Want to conceive		14 (21.2%)	52 (78.8%)
	Examination before pregnant		8 (12.1)	58 (87.9%)
	Family/ Relatives/Friends/Employer		6 (9.1%)	60 (90.9%)
	Influence			
	There are symptoms of cervical cancer		4 (6.1%)	62 (93.9%)
	Family history of cervical cancer		3 (4.5%)	63 (95.5%)
	Death of the family/relatives/ friends		3 (4.5%)	63 (95.5%)
	caused by cervical cancer			
	Others		2 (3.0%)	64 (97.0%)

Cross-tabulation analysis was done to determine the contribution factors that direct these women did the PST. As we can see, out of 66 women who did the PST, most of them, 52 (78.8%) did for detection of cervical cancer, 43 (65.2%) did for health purpose, 29 (43.9%) did because being advised by doctor, and 17 (25.8%)did as examination after delivery. 14 (21.2%) of the women did the PST due to examination for getting conceive, and 8 (12.1%) did as examination before pregnant. Only 6 women (9.1%) did the test as influenced from the family, relatives, friend or employer. Similarly, only 4 (6.1%) of them have the symptoms of cervical cancer. and about 3 (4.5%) did since they have the family history of cervical cancer. Alike, there are about 3 (4.5%) of these women did because they have experienced death of the family, relatives or friends caused by cervical cancer. And also, 2 (3.0%) of them have their own reasons which includes pathological conditions such as appearance of tumour.

Table 4.2.2: The barriers that prevented women doing the PST.

Have you undergone PST?	Reasons	Yes	No
No			
Count/%			
	Don't know/ Never heard about PST	47 (61.8%)	29 (38.2%)
	Don't know where to get the PST	22 (28.9%)	54 (71.1%)
76	Don't have time/ busy	16 (21.1%)	60 (78.9%)
100%	Fear	14 (18.4%)	62 (81.6%)
	Think it is not important	11 (14.5%)	65 (85.5%)
	Embarrassment	11 (14.5%)	65 (85.5%)
	No encouragement from Husband/	10 (13.2%)	66 (86.8%)
	Family/ Friends		
	Painful	7 (9.2%)	69 (90.8%)
	Expansive	6 (7.9%)	70 (92.1%)
	Pap smear makes me worry	5 (6.6%)	71 (93.4%)
	Don't care	4 (5.3%)	72 (94.7%)
	No female doctor	3 (3.9%)	73 (96.1%)
	Distant Hospital/ Clinic	3 (3.9%)	73 (96.1%)
	Loss of virginity	3 (3.9%)	73 (96.1%)
	Against your Religion/Culture/ Principe	0 (0.0%)	76(100.0%)
	Others	2 (2.6%)	74 (97.4%)

The table above shows the barriers that prevents these women from undergo the PST. There are about 76 women who never do the PST and among all, which is about most of them 47 (61.8%), don't know or never heard about PST before, while 22 (28.9%) of them don't know where to get the PST. Busy or don't have time, fear, thinks it is not important and embarrassment reported with 16 (21.1%), 14 (18.4%), 11 (14.5%), and 11 (14.5%) respectively. 10 (13.2%) of these women didn't receive the test due to no encouragement from their husband, family or friends. Feeling of painful, expensive, and pap smear will make them worry, constitutes with 7 (9.2%), 6 (7.9%), and 5 (6.6%) each. About 4 (5.3%) of these women don't care about the test. 3 (3.9%) each, of women reported that no female doctor, distant hospital or clinic and loss of virginity are among their reasons for rejecting the test. However, there are 2 (2.6%) of the women have their own reasons such as they did the appointment but not being called and they are not ready yet.

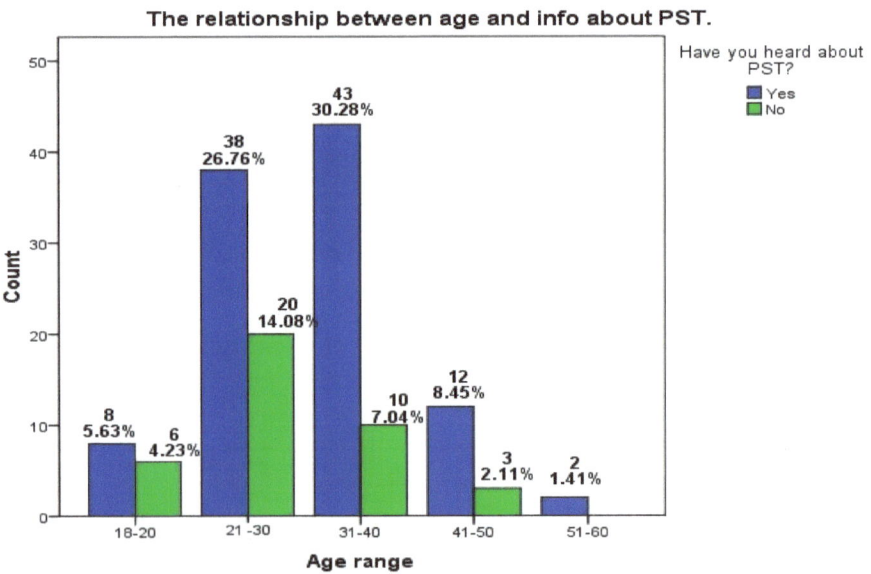

Figure 4.2.1: The relationship between age and info about PST

According to this figure, the women who heard about PST mostly between 31 to 40 years old which gives 30.28%, and women between 21 to 30 years old placed the second most. Whereas the lowest number of women who heard about it are elderly which aged between 51 to 60 years with 1.41%.

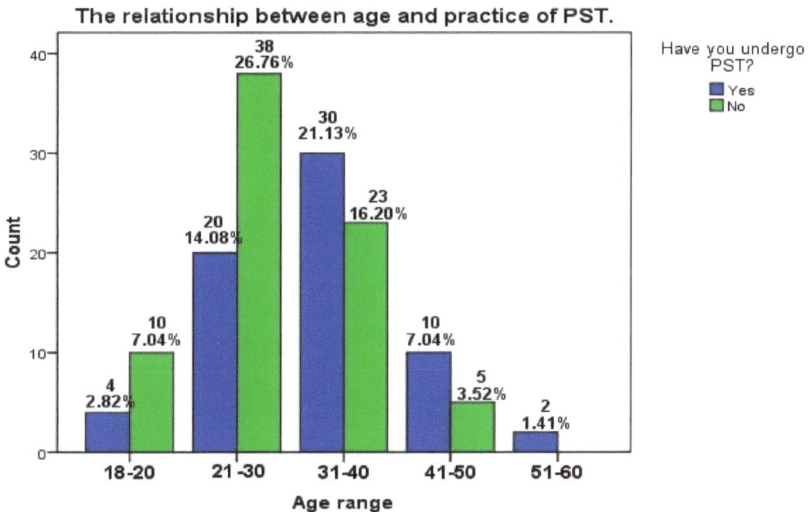

Figure 4.2.2: The relationship between age and practice of PST

This figure shows the relationship between age of the respondents with the practice of PST. The most frequent women who practice the PST are about 31 to 40 years old which constitutes 21.13% and the least age that practice the test is between 51 to 60 years old with 1.41%. Contritely, most women who are aged between 21 and 30 years old did not practice the PST which constitutes the highest percentage with 26.76%.

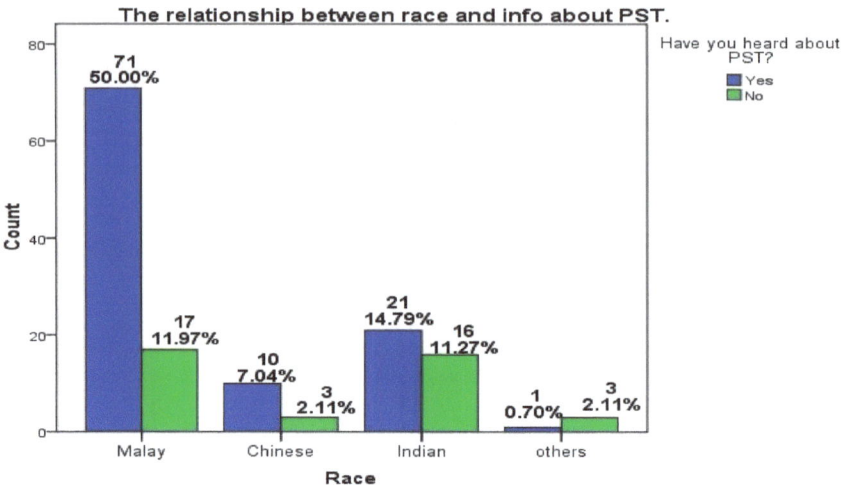

Figure 4.2.3: The relationship between race and info about PST

Among multiracial respondents who participated, majority of the Malay with about 50% have heard about the PST, and second most are Indian with 14.79%, followed with Chinese 7.04% and others (Sabah and Sarawak) with 0.70%.

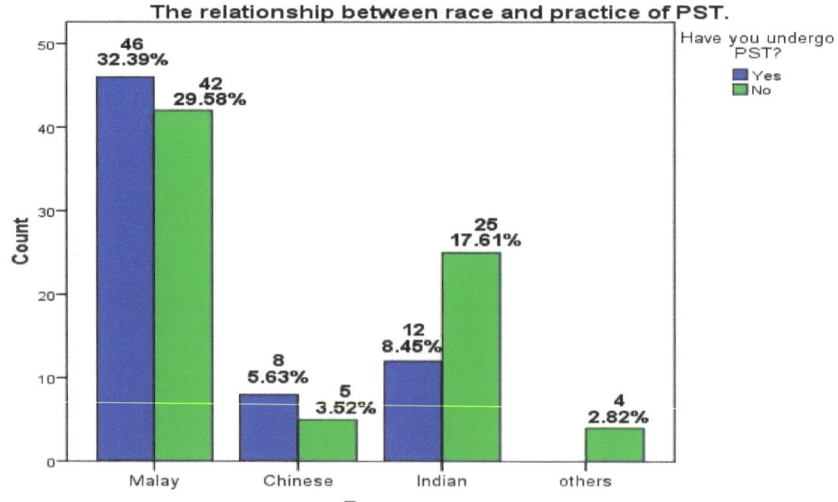

Figure 4.2.4: Race and the practice of PST

Among these multiracial groups, 32.4% of Malay practices PST, followed by 8.45% Indian, and 5.63% Chinese.

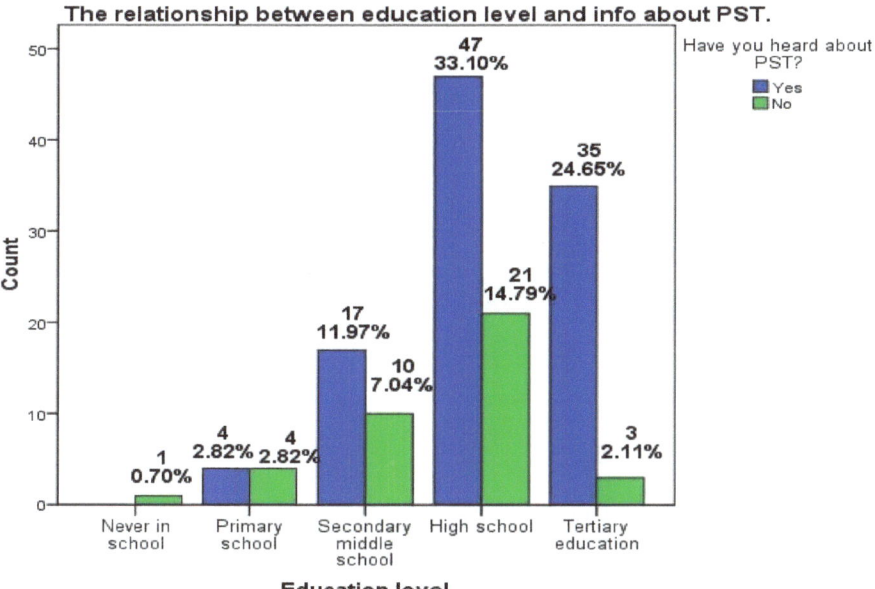

Figure 4.2.5: The relationship between education level and info about PST

The highest respondents with 33.10% who have heard about PST were the high school leavers, and respondents who graduated from tertiary education placed in the second with 24.65%. About 0.70% of the women who never been in school never heard about PST.

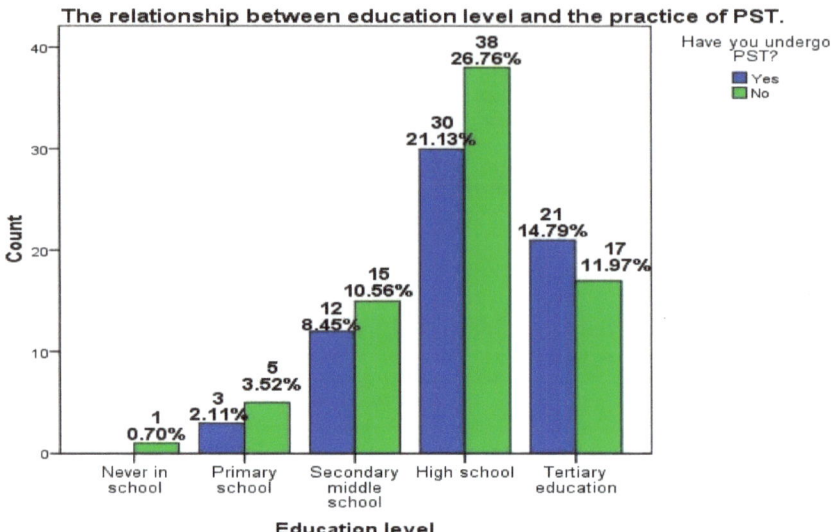

Figure 4.2.6: The relationship between education level and the practice of PST

Similar with the previous figure, high school leaver practice the most with 21.13%, second most are the women who graduated from tertiary education and women who never been in school never do the PST.

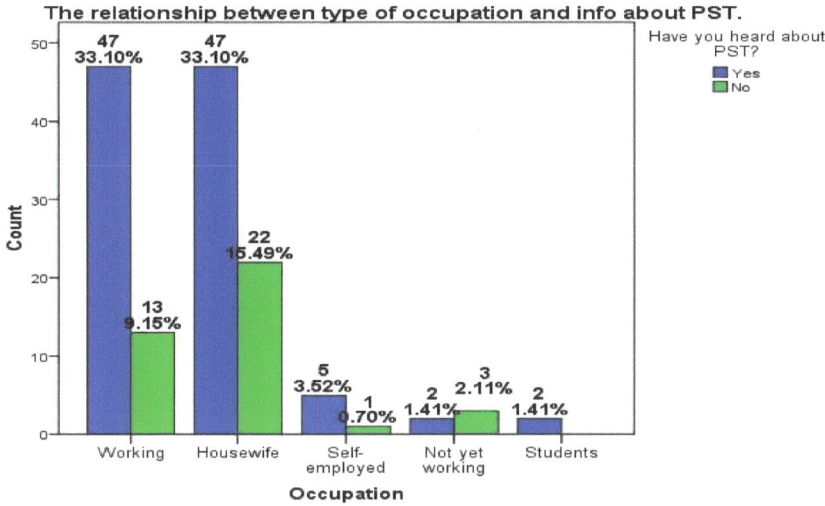

Figure 4.2.7: The relationship between type of occupation and info about PST

The women, who are working and being a housewife, both have heard about PST. They shared the same percentage with 33.10%. Both, women who are not working and currently students also contribute about 1.41% respectively.

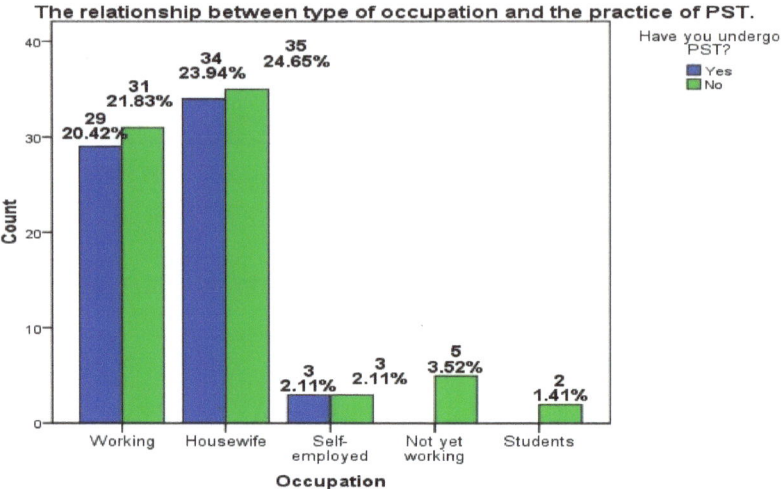

Figure 4.2.7: The relationship between type of occupation and the practice of PST

Impressively, among these women, housewife contributes the highest percent of person who practice the PST with 23.94%, and working women placed second with 20.42%. The women who are not practice the PST are women who are not working and the students.

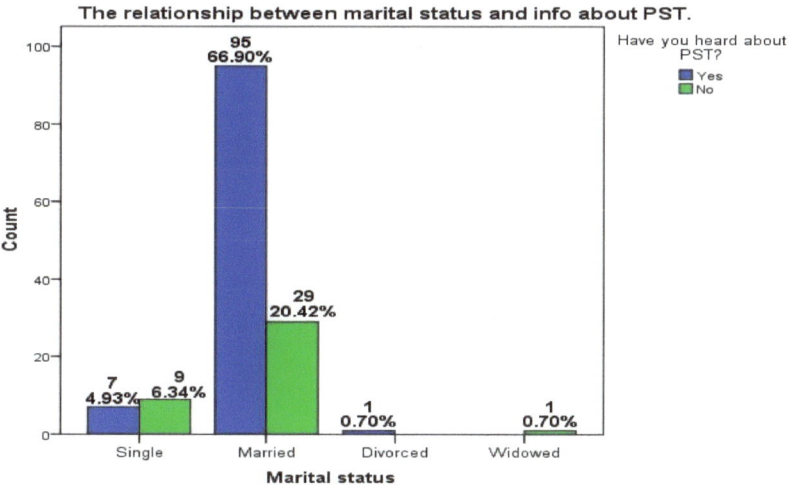

Figure 4.2.9: The relationship between marital status and information about PST

66.9% of the women who practice the PST were married, while only 4.9% are single.

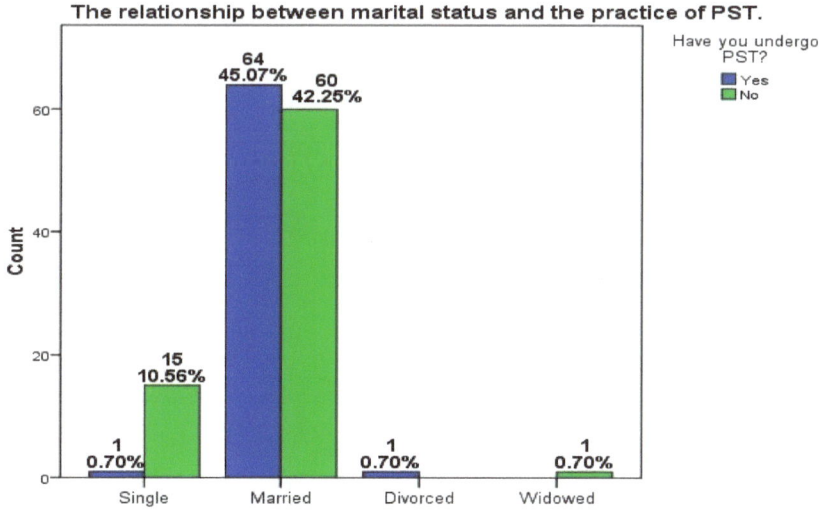

Figure 4.2.10: The relationship between marital status and practice of PST

As expected, most of the women who did the PST were married with 45%, while the single and divorced women shared the same of 0.70%.

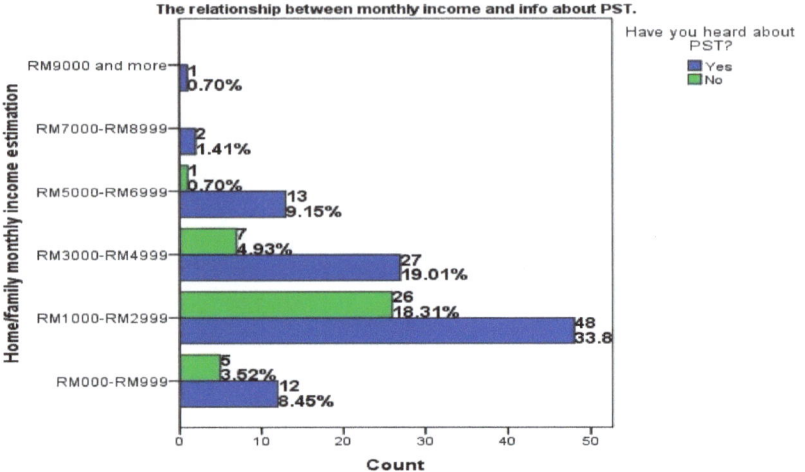

Figure 4.2.11: The relationship between monthly income and PST information

Most of the women who have heard about PST are with family income ranged between 1000-2999RM with 33.8%. Never the less, women who came from family with less income heard the least.

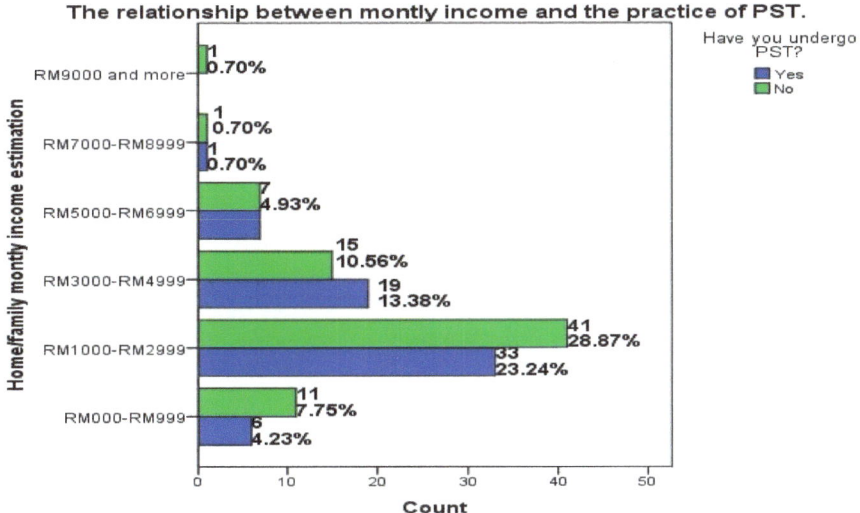

Figure 4.2.12: The relationship between income and PST practice

This figure illustrates that the highest women (23.24%) who practices the PST are women came from moderate family income.

4 CURRENT SITUATION

The selection of hospital in this study was not representative of the Malaysia women as a whole; moreover the number of participating respondents in the clinics was small relative to the total number in the hospital. The women respondents in the study were all randomly selected; large proportions were volunteers, and as such, this sample was not statistically representative of all women in Malaysia. Voluntary participation would have led to a bias for greater inclusion of women who were more health conscious, or with a greater propensity to seek information of their own health; while women who felt that they had less free time to spare could have been less likely to volunteer. In the clinic where researcher had to rely on volunteers doing the study in their own time, the participation rate was generally low which took a longer time to accomplish the sample data.

In spite of the weakness outlined above, this study is an important one because of the lack of research in Malaysia on the Pap smear screening practice among Malaysia women in general and out patients in O&G clinic in particular. Although not statistically representative of the whole Malaysia women, the current study provides data from a relatively large number of Malaysian women that could be compared with, thereby making its contribution to the existing literature.

The prevalence of practice of the Pap Smear Test (PST) among Malaysian women.

Based on figure 4.1.2; The rate of ever having had a Pap smear among Malaysian women in this study is nearly half with about 46.48% while on the other hand, 53.52% 43 of the women never had a Pap smear in their life. This is a relatively low as can be expected from our hypothesis which is the practice is high among women who visited the O&G clinic at Tengku Ampuan Rahimah Hospital. Similar finding by (Udigure, 2000) reported low levels of practicing the Pap Smear Test is 5-7% amongst female health workers. Contrary, (Yu & Rymer, 2003) found that of the respondents (650), 80.5% had had at least one smear test and 71.5% of these women have regular smears. (Allahverdipour & Emami, 2008) on a similar study with a total of 333 married women of childbearing age were recruited with cluster sampling, a total of 68.5% reported having undergone at least one

Pap test. In the same line, (Harlan et al. 1991) in a study conducted by 15 state health departments and the Distrct of Columbia, reported that 72% of the female participants had a Pap smear within the last year. The factors that affecting the practice of PST will be further discussed later.

Remarkably, among these women, the highest frequency of doing the practice at period was 15 times with 0.7% and majority of the respondent with 23.24% did the PST once at time of study. Most of these women did their first PST after the delivery (28.17%), second most (9.86%) after married and (7.04%) after experiencing bleeding or discharge. Others which are 1.41% of the respondents did the test during pregnancy and after a year on contraceptive pills intake. They seem to be well aware about the function of the PST. This is because the obstetric patient should receive a PST at her first prenatal visit as part of her initial evaluation. The cytological findings of those smears in this particular group of women have been the subject of extensive research since the 1960s. This research has generally focused on the following areas: 1) the ability to accurately diagnose preneoplastic lesions during pregnancy in light of the numerous diagnostic pit falls that result from the physiologic changes occur during pregnancy, 2) the use of hormonal evaluation and maturity index to predict fetal status, e.g., maturation, sex, placental activity, or an inevitable abortion, 3) the detection of the significance of inflammation and infectious agents (Michael, 1999).

The Practice of PST and the reasons why.

Amongst 66 women who practice the PST in our study, the reason of 78.8% of them did the test is for detection of cervical cancer. This is coinciding with the function of PST as the most successful screening test for carcinoma in the history of medicine. Its main benefit is the early detection of preneoplastic lesions. This indicates that Malaysian women in this clinic were aware of the Cervical Cancer and its preventive measures. The utilization of the PST for early detection of cervical cancer is better established, although the reliability of the test varies and is dependent on the expertise of the health professionals who take the smear as well as those who examine it (Chee et al. 2003b). (Wang & Lin, 1996) found that a substantial proportion (91.7%) of women were of the attitude that cancer can be treated if detected early enough.

Based on specific cytologic criteria, the diagnoses of candida, trichomonas, herpes simplex virus and human papilloma virus can be reliably rendered on Pap smears. Although Clamydia trochomatis and gonococcal species cannot be accurately diagnosed on Pap smears due to the lack of specific cytologic features, they are frequently associated with inflammatory exudates and reactive cellular changes. Inflammation by itself on Pap smears is not necessarily indicative of infection, and an inflammatory component is commonly seen on Pap smears from pregnant women (Michael, 1999). This is the reason why 65.2% of women in our study did the PST for the health purpose. They account for the second higher reasons. Studies in other countries have also found a close association between PST and health care utilization indicator. In the Singapore community-based study, interestingly found that women were more likely to have had the last smear as a self-initiated screening test or part of a regular health check-up rather than as part of a postnatal or family planning visit. (Chee et al. 2003b).

When they investigates the effects of potential barriers and facilitators of screening by one's own physician given no symptoms, they found that the barrier of fear getting cancer was associated with a greater likelihood of having PST (Kressin et al. 2010).
About 43.9% from these women did the PST due to advice from the doctors or physicians. Without a doubt, health care providers influence women's screening behaviours. It is proved in a study by (Wong et al. 2008) which found that underutilization of cervical cancer screening may be due in part of lack of physician's recommendation. However, there is a need to improve patient-provider communication as women reported that they had

never been informed of the existence and importance of Pap smears by health care professionals. (Kressin et al. 2010) also stated that physician encouragement has associated with the likelihood to get screening. However Malaysian doctors has carried out their duties to deliver the information and educates the patients about PST, yet, it should be done with a broader prospective.

25.8% of these women did the test as a check-up routine after delivery or post-partum. This is consistent with gynaecologist recommendation that the women should do their Pap smear between six and eight weeks after delivery. The reason for waiting is that the test might otherwise show any inflammatory process that took place after birth, rather than true abnormalities of the cells. Post-partum check-up is important to assess any unusual inflammatory that might be happening. Londo et al. found that the postpartum Pap smears provide a higher yield of endocervical cells and better prediction of dysplasia than prepartum smears. Nonetheless, this does not lessen the importance of the initial smear, since a high number of these patients may be lost to follow-up through noncompliance (Michael, 1999).

Among other reasons are; 21.2% of the women did it because of intention to get pregnant and 12.1% did as an examination before getting pregnant. From these reasons we can determine that these women have knowledge to do medical tests to evaluate their reproductive health. This is because, for an instance; women with HIV are at greater risk of developing cervical cancer and other cervical abnormalities. (Michael, 1999) stated that since patients with sexually transmitted disease (STD) have a higher risk of preterm delivery and fetal morbidity, it is important to evaluate whether inflammation and/or the reactive changes caused by inflammation on Pap smears can reliably predict the presence of STD, particularly in asymptomatic patients. They found these patients to be at higher risk for STD and pregnancy-related complication. 46

Mean while, there are 9.1% of the women did the test due to influence from family and people surrounding, 6.1% and 4.5% did because of having the cervical cancer symptoms and family history respectively. Alike, there are about 4.5% of these women did because they have experienced death of the family, relatives or friends caused by cervical cancer. And also, 3.0% of them have their own reasons which include pathological conditions such as appearance of tumour. People influences have been proved to increase the PST rates. Other than people surrounding such as relatives, friends or employer, family is the most important one. Mother's role modelling has been shown to have a tremendous influence over a child's health care behaviour (Mattila et al. 2000). This was also shown in Vietnamese-American women (Tang, et al. 1999). Having a mother or family member that has had a Pap smears done and was willing to discuss this issue contributed to the uptake of PST (Wong et al. 2008). From this study we identify that self-conscious about the symptoms of cervical cancer affecting one's decisions. (Dunn et al. 2009) in their study stated that intuition would tend to suggest that individuals who have a history of illness will have had increased opportunities of interacting with the health care system and would thus be exposed to information regarding cervical cancer or PST. They also found that family history of illness exhibit a strong positive association with recent testing that is driven almost entirely by the Chinese, whereby an individual with a history of illness associated with a 22% increase in the probability of receiving a PST in the previous 3 years.

The Barriers of PST and the preventive factors.

After analysed the results, the majority of the women (77) out of total respondent did not have had a Pap smears before thus rejecting our hypotheses. Similar findings in Taiwan by (Wang & Lin 1996), found that 40% of the women have never had a PST and 86% have not had one in the past year. To investigate more about the reasons, we have identified the reasons that being selected by the respondents for not undergo the screening.

We found that more than half of these women don't know or never heard about PST before which accounts for 61.8%. This is such an interesting figure since this study was done in the O&G clinic where they can easily access to the information. However, this is not really surprising since we found the same situation in similar studies. They found that healthcare providers influence women's screening behavior. It was found that the underutilization of cervical cancer screening might be due to in part to a lack of physician recommendation. There appears to be a need to improve health education by healthcare provider, as women reposted that they had never been informed of the existence and importance of Pap smear by healthcare professionals (Wong et al. 2009). Similar in a research by (Dunn et al. 2009), they found that the most common reason was "Don't know", though interpreting what this response captures is complicated since respondents may have selected this for a number of reasons. A respondent may be signalling that they did not know what a PST was; they did not know that a PST was a recommended procedure, or they did not know why they had not received one.

Interestingly, the second most common reason reported by these 28.9% women is that they don't know where to get the PST. Another important barrier mentioned by the participants was lack of information about screening sites (Al-Naggar et al. 2010). (Abot Chie & Shokar, 2009) also reports the same finding. In parallel, (Ayinde et. al., 2004) found that 16% of their study participants had lack of knowledge of centres where the test could be done. Similar finding was reported by (Aniebue & Aniebue, 2010) reported that 34% of their participants did not know where to obtain a Pap smears. The places of screening should be easily addressed with simple information provision.

Thirdly, 21.1% of the respondents stated that they don't have time or too busy to do the PST. Similarly, (Wong et al., 2008) also found that one-third of their respondents value their own health as secondary to family and social responsibilities. In studies done in other Asian regions (Nguyen et al. 2004; Dabash et al. 2005) found that, many saw their daily domestic chores and family needs as more important than prevention of illness. Barriers such as having to take time off for screening, inconvenient schedule, and long time waiting time at the clinic all add up to their reluctance to have 48

Pap smears. Some other reasons that contributing to being too busy is might be to their work and time limitation. (Dunn et al. 2009) also found that amongst those who report "No time" as a reason for non-screening, each additional year of education increases the probability of having no time to being a reason for non-screening by 2%. This is likely due to the fact that females with higher levels of education are more likely to be in the labour force. (Williams et al. 2003) also supporting this statement since lack of time was cited as the most common reason (93%) for noncompliance among their respondents.

Fear accounts about 18.4% of the reason why these women did not go for the screening. Since they only choose "Fear", there is no further elaboration which can determine what these women are fear to. This is due to lack of additional explaining of the answer on the choices given. However we assume that these women might be fear of the procedural of how PST is done. (Harlan et al. 1991) their interview survey data of Cervical cancer screening: who is not screened and why? Also found that fear is most reason for non-compliance among their respondents. And (Williams et al. 2003) found that 14% of the women feel fear in seeing a doctor prevents them from receiving the PST. Alike, in the studies of (Bener et al. 2001; Maaita & Barakat 2002; Gamarra et al. 2005) reported that the fear of discovery of cancer is one of the barriers among study participants.

Among other reason for non-screening is 14.5% of the women think that Pap smear is not important to them. Our finding is consistence with (Wong et al. 2008) which in their studies provide an insight into the beliefs and attitudes of Malaysian women with respect to why they do not go for screening. It also parallels with other studies (Jirowong et al. 1994; Maaita & Barakat 2002; Holroyd et al. 2004; Islam et al. 2006) that woman's attitudes and beliefs influenced screening behaviours. Many women expressed a lack of personal susceptibility to cervical cancer and therefore believed it to be unnecessary to do Pap smear. According to theory of illness behaviour, such self-perceptions could be related to the underlying distinction between "self-defined" versus "other-defined" illness (Scambler 2004). In line with this, (Wang & Lin 1996) found that overall 76.2% of their respondents perceived the disease to be a common one and 32.6% of the respondents thought the age group 40s and 50s to be the most affected by cervical cancer. This type of perception has leads to non-compliance among women. In addition, (Yu & Rymer 2003) also found that women had a positive attitude to cervical cancer screening but as long as they felt healthy, they chose not to attend. Similar in (Ackerson & Greteback, 2007) noted, intrinsic motivators were related to beliefs and perceptions of vulnerability, such as ignoring cervical cancer screening when no symptoms were present; believing that not knowing if one had cervical cancer was better; and thinking that only women who engage in sexual risk-taking behaviours need to obtain PST. (Harlan et al. 1991) also found that the largest category of reasons given by women for being non-compliant was they believed it was unnecessary, had no problems, or had been procrastinating.

Embarrassment was reported as barriers for about 14.5% of these women. Similar studies reported that included embarrassment was the barriers among the participants (Bener et al. 2001; Maaita & Brakat 2002; Gamarra et al. 2005). Embarrassment was confirmed by other reports (Ganguly 1995; Lovell et al. 2007). However, we cannot determine what are the exact reasons that causing these women to embarrass. We assume that these women are embarrassed if people know that they do the screening or embarrass towards the healthcare personnel during the procedure. (Dunn et al. 2009) in their studies found that, there are different perceptions within these women. Individuals who live in rural communities are 12% more likely to report being embarrassed for non-screening compared to their urban cohort. This may also result from differing amounts of exposure to medical practice or even the presence of cultural taboos between urban and rural residents. Equally (Yu & Rymer 2003) also found the perceived barriers such as embarrassment played a part in women's decision in returning for regular smear. (Kahn et al. 1999) also reported that embarrassment was associated with having a stranger examine one's body or having a male provider performed a pelvic examination.

13.2% of these women had chosen no encouragement husband, family or friends to do the test as the barriers. There are some studies that supporting our finding. (Abotchie & Shokar 2009) reported that one of the barriers among their study participants that whether their partner would want them to have a PST. And in (Kahn et. al. 1999) reported that peers advising them against having a PST was a barrier. While on the 50 other hand, the positive influence of physician recommendation on cancer screening uptake has been well documented in numerous studies in the United States (Burnett et al. 1995; Nguyen et al. 2002). This is show that, encouragement from the people around is also important in influencing one's decision of taking a PST.

An expectation of pain and discomfort during the procedure was another barrier reported by 9.2% of these women. This is supported by (Wong et al. 2008) in their studies. Stigmatization of pelvic examinations among their respondent was a result of exposure to sensationalized anecdotes or "medical gossip" by peers. Perceived pain as described by peers appeared to be a great barrier to participation in screening. It has been reported that such exchange of personal health information among lay people played an important role in lay referral system in health care (Suls & Goodkin 1994). Similar study reported that included misconception about the test being painful were among the participants (Bener et al. 2001; Maaita & Brakat 2002; Gamarra et al. 2005). This may be a difficult barrier to overcome among asymptomatic women. Those who expressed this concern may have had painful and unpleasant experiences with prior to PST, or have heard about such experience from others. While in the study of (Kahn et al. 1999), the respondents who agreed with these barriers reported frequently that pain or discomfort was associated with provider behaviour or style. For instance, one adolescent linked lack of education or preparation for the examination with pain, explaining that, "the pain [and] the uncertainty...goes hand in hand". Similarly, several adolescent reported that pain could be minimized if the examination was performed in a gentle manner. Comments also revealed that many adolescents believe the pelvic examination to be a remarkably negative experience.

Another barriers reported by these women is expensive with about 7.9% of the women supports this reason. (Al-Naggar et al. 2010) found that cost is one of the important barriers reported by almost half of the participants. There are similar finding that was reported by (Ayinde et al. 2004) that 5.9% of their participants mentioned that the cost is one of the barriers of PST. However, refer to the above mentioned, what surprising us is that this study is done in the government hospital and government already subsidized the PST and women can do this test for free. This kind of perception might be given by women who did not update the current health care information.

6.6% of these women reported that PST will cause them worry. Even though it is relatively low, however it is still the important barriers. In studies by (Kahn et al. 1999), they found that 11 participants reported fear of the finding a problem and fear of the unknown. Several explained that they would feel unclean or blame themselves if they were told that they had STD or an abnormal Pap smear. "Denial or invincibility" was reported by 6 participants, several of whom describes the belief that if abnormalities were left alone, they would eventually disappear. Similar findings found in (Oscarsson et al. 2008) which stated that fear of the results also influenced their non-attendance.

A relatively small number of women (5.3%) reported that they do not care of the PST as the barriers. Does not care here mean that, they do not concern about the existence of cervical cancer screening. This also been reported by (Kahn et al. 1999) that 4 out of 15 respondents reported that; the not wanting to look for trouble was a barrier. This negative attitude should be changed in order to increase the screening rates.

The absence of female doctor reported for about 3.9% and is not very alarming. This indicates that women nowadays are more open about the health care system. However, it is still an important barrier that if not being prevented, can reduce the rates of screening. Several previous studies also revealed that women reported high levels of embarrassment and anxiety about having vaginal or pelvic examination by male doctors. Due to religious affiliation and cultural beliefs, Muslim women in particular felt most comfortable with female health care providers. Many of them did not participate in screening due to perceived unavailability of female doctors (Wong et al. 2008) This is consistent with other research with Asian women, as many studies reported that they preferred female doctors to perform physical examination on intimate body parts and were highly embarrassed with male health providers (Nguyen et al. 2000; Holroyd et al. 2004).

Distant hospitals or clinics are the barriers reported from 3.9% of these women. The absence of the nearest health care provider seems to prevent them from doing the PST. (Kresin et al. 2010) also stated that having screening nearby has association with agreater willingness to be screened. Hence, providing the easy access of getting a PST might solve this problem. Lastly, losing of virginity also prevent 3.9% of these women from being screened. Even though, PST is not being recommended towards unmarried women, this barrier indicates that these women might due to lack of knowledge in this regard and may be due to cultural and the background of the respondent. (Al-Naggar et al. 2010) also found that nearly half of their study participants mentioned that PST will affect their virginity. Similar finding was reported by (Abotchie & Shokar 2009).

Pap Smear Test Knowledge.

Regarding the knowledge evaluation in our study, we did not have the specific assessment to measures one's knowledge and there is no statistic data since it is difficult to claim their overall knowledge. Nevertheless, we believe that these qualitative results are still informative and significant. Three aspects of knowledge which contributed significantly were; 1) Purpose of the test, 2) the frequency and the target women, and 3) risk factors towards cervical cancer.

From our study, we found that 72.54% of these women have heard about Pap smear screening test in their lives. However, having heard is not necessary indicates that they know what is the PST is about. This statistic data is relatively high as we expect in our hypothesis that women in the O&G should have more information about this screening test since they have the easy access to the doctors or the hospital/clinics in directly. Alike, (Harlan et al. 1991) also found that in their study, only 0.2 % of the women had never heard of PST.

Majority of these women (57.7%) have heard about PST from their doctor, hospital or from clinic. This is really satisfying. Second most popular sources are from the printed media such as news paper, magazine, books, flyers and etc with 43.7%. The third place is from the electronic media such as television and radio, and the least is from the workplace or the employer. We assume that the workplace of these women is varying according to the suitability. (Makinuddin & Ali 1997) stated that they found satisfactory dissemination of information on cervical cancer were acquired from radio, television, newspaper and staff nurses were associated with high level of knowledge on cervical cancer. Even though, health care worker is the primary source of information, however nowadays we found that the government has started to realize this and many campaigns started to be viewed in the electronic media.

To extend the analysis, we want to be acquainted with whether women who have heard about the PST is actually know the purpose if they were screening for cervical cancer, and impressively 73.9% of them know that the purpose of the test. While only 2.1% said it is for detection of STD.

(Dunn et al. 2009) also found the same finding. This is congruent with the similar finding in the NHMS, where 86.6% of the women who had the test knew this reason for doing so (Chee et al. 2003b)

Majority of these women do not know how often should PST been done. However for those who knew, 38% said it should be done once a year and 18.3% said once in 1 to 3 years while the least of 1.4% chosen once in the 5 years. Even though, the choices given are all correct, we just want to determine the basic knowledge among these women. Official recommendation is for women to undergo the PST annually in the initial 2 years, and subsequently, once every 3 years, with priorities for sexually active women who are more than 35 years old, have more than 5 children, have practiced contraception for more than 5 years or who are new acceptors of family planning services, and women who diagnosed with STD. Women who attend postnatal and family planning services are primary targets. (Chee et al. 2003a) Similar study also found that women who were unfamiliar with the procedure were not queried. Of those familiar, 77.9% describe appropriate intervals as 13 to 36 months (one to three years) while 10.2% said annually (Harlan et al. 1991).

No women could be forced to get a Pap smear (Mc Gain & Hayloc, 2003), notwithstanding, 25.4% of these women opposing this fact. However, majority of these women agreeing with the fact that women cannot be forced to do the PST. In today's health-care system in the United States, as in many other countries, the responsibility for a person's health rests mainly with that person.

Regarding the opinion, 80.3% of women in our study agreed that married women should receive the PST. Despite the fact, about 77.5% and 76.8% of the women said that women who have the family history of cervical cancer and have its symptoms are the primary target too. Although the policy is to target all sexually active women, in practice, married women have more access due to a variety of reasons. One of the reasons is that is a recent policy change, and prior to 1995, when a nation-wide campaign on prevention of breast and cervical cancer was carried out, the official policy was to provide cervical cancer screening for married women only. (Chee et al. 2003b)

More than half of these women knew that the cervical cancer is caused by viral infection; nonetheless, the type of virus is not being stated. 66.2% is moderately low compare with those women who claimed that having heard about PST. Similar, (Wong et al. 2009) found that only 40% of the participants had previously heard about Human Papilloma Virus (HPV). Knowledge of Pap smear (96%) is higher than of HPV (41%). Subsequently, nearly half of these women (49.3%) knew that the infection is caused by sexual intercourse while the rest is not. The incidence of squamous intraepithelial lesion (SIL) is increasing among sexually active female especially those with sexually transmitted disease (STD) (Michael, 1999). On the whole, women appeared to be well informed of the link between the number of sexual partners and cervical cancer (Yu & Rymer, 2003).

Overall, knowledge about Pap smear is moderately low but still has potential to be improved. The majority of these women have heard about PST and majority of them knew its main purpose. However, the link between having heard, the practice and the risk factors toward cervical cancer are still poor.

Attitude Towards Pap smear Test.

This study also analysed the attitude of the women. From here we found that 44.37% (or 82.89% among of the women who never had a PST) have the intention to be screened in the near future. While 16.9% (31.58% from never had PST) of these women not sure exactly when they want to be screened, and 15.49% (28.9% from 55 never had PST) will do it after get a doctor's consultation. 9.15% (17.1% from never had PST) give the negative attitude of persisting rejecting the screening test. (Harlan et al. 1991) similarly found that in England, a general medical practice studied women overdue for PST. Of the 118 women personally contacted, 47% said they had no major objection to the test, but it was of low priority. Another 24% gave reasons for not having the procedure which were based on incorrect information and 29% had strong objections to the test and would probably never consult to having the PST. Impressively, majority of 73.24% of women in our study would like to encourage other women to do the screening. These positive attitudes are noteworthy in increasing the PST screening rates in the future.

The Relationship of Practice and Sociodemographic.

In this study there is relationships between having heard and practice regarding with socio-demographic factors. From here we found that the women who having heard and did the PST is highest in adult women between 31 to 40 years old, both with 30.28% and 21.13% respectively. And the least of among both is in the elderly between 51 to 60 years old, both with only 1.41%. Regarding the practice, young women is the highest in who did not get the screening yet which is between 21 to 30 years old with 26.76%. We believe that young women constitutes the highest might be due to unmarried and not aware of the importance of screening. Age is the strongest factor affecting PST use, particularly for women below age 30 and over the age of 65 (Wang & Lin, 1996). Similar studies supported our findings that there is a relationship between age and knowledge about cervical cancer screening. Another study also showed that age was associated with knowledge about PST (Maxwell et al. 2001) In terms of practice, the higher age of the women, the more they did the test, except for elderly who might think that PST is not for them. The Pap smear screening pattern was found to significantly increase with women younger than 35 years old and older than 30 years compare to elderly (Chee et al, 2003b). As well in (Kressin et al. 2010) also noted that in their bivariate analyses indicated that, older age is more associated with more willingness for cancer screening by one's own physician when there are no symptoms.

Although race has been associated with numerous negative predictors of cancer screening compared to other socio-demographic factors, race itself, are important driving force behind such associations, as has been found with regard to health care utilization in general. Among women who participate in our study, Malays constitutes the highest with 62%, Indian

26.1%, Chinese 9.2% and others is 4%. After analysed we found that among of these 3 races, the women who having heard and practice the PST is highest among Malays but this might be due unequally distributed of sample. When we studied these variables individually, we noticed that most of the Indian women with 56.76% among them have heard about PST but only 32.43% did the test. Malay who is the majority of the participants reported with 80.68% have heard about PST and only 52.27% undergo the screening. In the same line, 76.92% of Chinese women have heard about PST and 61.54% of them did the test. Thus among these, Malays is the top among women who have heard about PST, followed by Chinese and Indians. While, Chinese women is the highest regarding the practice, followed by Malays and Indians. Similar studies also found that ethnicity has a strong statistically significant effect on the propensity of undertaking PST. Compare to Malays, women who self-report Chinese are more likely to test for cervical cancer by 11%. In contrast, women who self-report Indian ethnicity are 19% less likely to go through PST compared to Malays (Dunn et al. 2009).

Given the suggestive format of the question, we interpret this is a clear sign that knowledge of cervical cancer and the necessary screening procedures are leaking in the Indian community.
Education levels are found to be influencing the knowledge and the PST practices. Our study revealed that the women who have heard about PST the most is the one who at least finished their high school with 33.1% and finished their tertiary education with 24.65%, while the women who were never in school never heard about it. Alike in the practice, women who finished the high school and tertiary education constitute the most with 21.12% and 14.79% respectively. As expected, the women who never in school or less than high school is the lowest. Our findings were supported by (Harlan et al. 1991) which stated that women with less than a high school education were 3 times as likely to have never heard of a Pap smear and women failing to complete high school were much more likely to be non-compliant with screening than those who graduated. Women with lower levels of education tend to underuse the Pap smear screening (Wang & Lin 1996).

Types of occupation were tested to be associated with the knowledge and practice of PST in our study. In our study, housewife and working women are equal among women who have heard about PST with 33.10% each. And for those who had practiced the test, housewife were slightly ahead with 23.94% compared with working women who with 20.42%. We assume time barrier is the preventive factors among working women. (Kahn et al. 1999) also reported that prolonged waiting time at the clinic, taking time off from school or work, finding child care, not having transportation, the clinic being too far away and not having time or energy to make appointment is among the reasons of not compliant. Some also stated that being employed was only associated with willingness for screening by one's physician when one has symptom (Kressin et al. 2010). Marital status seemingly predispose to the Pap smear screening. Our study exposed that married women is the leading regarding who have heard and did the PST with 66.9% and 45.07% compare to others. Divorced and widowed women are the least in this criterion. And only 4.93 % of single women have heard and 0.7% did the PST. Other Malaysian studies also show the dependence of Pap smear screening on marital status.

In the NHMS, only 2.7% of single women had ever had a Pap smear, compared to 33.4% married women, 18.3% divorced women, 9.1% widowed women, and 10.5% among women who were cohabiting (Chee et al. 2003a). Other study also ruled out that among staff members of a local university, Pap smear screening was also significantly associated with being married.

Income is also a predisposing factor affecting the screening. We found that, women with family monthly income between RM1000 to RM2999 were the highest in both have heard and practiced the PST with 33.8% and 23.24% each and those who are lesser than RM999 also less in practice. This is rather a moderate income for Malaysian. We also found that women who have monthly family income RM3000 and above are inversely proportional with the practice of PST. Individual with less income receive cancer screening less often than do those with higher level income (Kressin et al. 2010). Similar, they also found that with income level between $50,000 and $75,000 were less likely to be willing to have cancer screening by one's physician, compared to those of the highest income.

5 FUTURE DIRECTIONS

It can be concluded that the practice of the Pap smear Test among Malaysian women are moderate and the overall knowledge about the test is moderately low and there are significant relation between the practice and the sociodemographic factors. However, Malaysian women showing a positive attitude towards the screening test. The null hypothesis is approved and the objectives are reached.

There are many ways that the authority can do to increase the rate of practice since we already know what prevents these women from undergo the screening. Our findings suggest that public health officials must focus greater resources on educating women about cervical cancer and women's health issues to increase testing prevalence in the country. But we believe the real value of our analysis is how it informs the type of education campaigns that would be most effective for different groups within the country.

The campaigns could utilize various language based media such as; newpapers, popular magazines, television programs, radio channels or even famous celebrities or spoke persons form a particular ethnic group as a role model to highlight the benefits of PST screening. Practitioners have an opportunity to impact the incidence and mortality of cervical cancer by improving screening practice of minority women. They can emphasize the importance of obtaining pap smear regularly, teach patients the risks for and signs and symptoms of cervical cancer, and provide recommendations for obtaining screening at low cost to the patient. Developing trust, having a consistent provider, making the patient feel at ease, and being able to communicate well can encourage the women.

Moreover, reminders about the appointment-making may enhance the rates. Other than that, we are suggesting that expanded hours for the colposcopy clinic; avoiding long waits for an appointment, providing babysitting or transportation, and ensuring that a person 60 answers the telephone when a patient's call to make an appointment can enhance the appointment. We found that formal education had a positive association with the testing behaviour of females.

This suggests that programs to educate and create awareness amongst school girls may have a direct and positive impact in increasing the likelihood of participating in PST screening. Recent announcements that Malaysia is introduce a program to vaccinate all 13-year old girls against cervical cancer in 2010 is potentially a positive step towards achieving this objective, since information about the need for PST screening throughout their adult lives could be incorporated into the vaccination program.

REFERENCES

Ab. Karim, B., & (MS, 2008) Abd. Latip, K. (1997). Knowledge and Perception Towards Pap Smear Among Women Who Visited Health Clinics in Kuala Terengganu District, 1997. *Community Health Journal*, 12 (1).

Abotchie PN, Shokar NK (2009). Cervical cancer screening among college students in ghana: knowledge and health beliefs. *Int J Gynecol Cancer*, 19, 412-6.

Ackerson, K., & Greteback, K. (2007). Factors Influencing Cancer Screening Pratices of Underserved Women. *J Am Acad Nurse Pract*, 19(11): 591-601.

Allahverdipour, H., & Emami, A. (2008). Perception of Cervical Cancer Threat, Benefits, and Barriers of Papanicolaou Smear Screening Program For Women In Iran. *Women Health*, 47 (3): 23-37.

Al-Naggar, R.A., Low, W.Y., & Md Isa, Z. (2010). Knowledge and Barriers Towards Cervical Cancer Screening Among Young Women in Malaysia. Asian Pacific J Cancer Prev, . 11: 867-873.

Aniebue PN, Aniebue UU (2010). Awareness and practice of cervical cancer screening among female undergraduate students in a Nigerian university. *J Cancer Educ*, 25, 106-8.

Ayinde OA, Omigbodun AO, Ilesanmi AO (2004). Awareness of cervical cancer, papanicolaou's smear and its utilisation among female undergraduates in ibadan. *Afr J Reprod Hlth*. 8, 68-80.

Badrinath, P., Ghazal-Aswad, S., Deemas, E., & McIlvenny, S. (2004). A Study of Knowledge, Attitude, and Practice of Cervical Cancer Screening Among Female Primary Care Physician In The United Arab Emirates. *Health Care for Women International*, 25: 663-670.
Bener A, Denic S, Alwash R (2001). Screening for cervical cancer among Arab women (brief communication). *Int J Gynecol Obstet*, 74, 305-7.

Bourne, P. A., Charles, C. A., Francis, C. G., South-Bourne, N., & Peters, R. (2010). Perception, attitude and practices of women towards pelvic examination and pap smear in Jamaica. *North American Journal of Medical Sciences*, 2(10).

Burnett CB, Steakley CS, Tefft MC (1995). Barriers to breast and cervical cancer screening in underserved women in the district of columbia. *Oncol Nurs Forumm*, 22, 1551-7.

Charakorn, C., Rattanasiri, S., Lertkhachonsuk, A. A., Thanapprapasr, D., Chittithaworn, S., & Wilailak, S. (2011). Knowledge of Pap Smear, HPV and62 The HPV Vaccine and The Acceptability of The HPV Vaccine by Thai Women. *Asia Pac J Clin Oncol*, 7 (2): 160-7.

Chee, H. L., Rashidah, S., Shamsuddin, K., & Sharifah Zainiyah, S. Y. (2003a). Knowledge and Practice of Brest Self Examination and Pap Smear Screening Among a Group of Electronics Women Workers. *Med J Malaysia*, 58 (3): 320-329.

Chee, H. L., Rashidah, S., Shamsuddin, K., & Intan, O. (2003b). Factors Related To The Practice of Breast Self Examination (BSE) and Pap Smear Screening Among Malaysian Women Workers in Selected Electronics Factories. *BMC Women Health*, 3:3.

Dabash, R., Vajpayee, J., Jacob, M., Dzuba, I., Lal, N., Bradley, J., et al. (2005). A strategic assessment of cervical cancer prevention and treatment services in 3 districts of Uttar Pradesh, India. *Reproductive Health, 2*, 11.

Dunn, R. A., Tan, A. K., & Samad, M. I. (n.d). Why Women Do Not Get Screened For Cervical Cancer: Evidence From Malaysia. *Women Health-Malaysia*, Pages 0-26.

Gamarra, C. J., Paz, E. P., & Griep, R. H. (2005). Knowledge, Attitudes, and Practice Related To Papanicolaou Smear Test Among Argentina's Women. *Rev Saude Publica*, 39 (2) : 1-6.

Ganguly I (1995). Promoting the health of women of non-English speaking backgrounds in Australia. *World Hlth Forum*, 16, 157-63.
Guidebook for Pap Smear Screening, Ministry of Health, Kuala Lumpur: Division of Family Health Development, Ministry of Health Malaysia, 2004:1-2.

Harlan, L. C., Berbstein, A.B., & Kessler, L. G. (1991). Cervical Cancer Screening: Who Is Not Screened and Why? *American Journal of Public Health*, 81 (7): 885-890.

Hawkins, N. A., Cooper, C. P., Saraiya, M., Gelb, C. A., & Polonec, L. (2002). Why The Pap Test? Awareness and Use of The Pap Test Among Women in The United States. *Journal of Women's Health*.

Holroyd, E., Twinn, S.,&Adab, P. (2004). Social-cultural influences on Chinese women's attendance for cervical screening. *Journal Advance Nursing, 46*, 42–52.

Islam, N., Kwon, S. C., Senie, R., & Kathuria, N. (2006). Breast and cervical cancer screening among South Asian women in New York City. *Journal of Immigrant and Minority Health, 8*, 211–221.63.

Jirojwong, S., Thassri, J., & Skolnik M. (1994) Perception of illness and the use of health care givers among cervical cancer patients at Songkla Nagarind Hospital. A study in southern Thailand. *Cancer Nursing, 17*, 395–402.
Kahn, J. A., Chiou, V., Allen, J. D., Goodman, E., Perlman, S. E., & Emans, S. J. (1999). Beliefs About Papanicolaou Smears and Compliance With Papanicolaou Smear Follow-up in Adolescents. *American Medical Association*, 1046-1054.

Kressin, N. R., Manze, M., Russell, S. L., Katz, R. V., Caludio, C., Green, B. L., et al. (2010). Self- reported Willingness To Have Cancer Screening and The Effect of Sociodemographic Factors. *J Natl Med Assoc*, 102(3): 219-27.

Lim GCC, Halimah Y, eds. Second Report of the National Cancer Registry. *Cancer, Incidence in Malaysia 2003*. Kuala Lumpur: National Cancer Registry, 2004.

Lovell S, Kearns RA, Friesen W (2007). Sociocultural barriers to cervical screening in South Auckland, New Zealand. *Soc Sci Med*, 65, 138-50.

Londo R, Bjelland T, Girod C, Glasser M. Prenatal and postpartum Pap smears: do we need both. Fam Pract Res J 1994; 14:359 367.
Maaita M, Brakat M (2002). Jordanian women's attitudes towards cervical cancer screening and cervical cancer. *J Obstet Gynecol*, 22, 421-2.

Makinuddin, A. A., & Ali, O. (1997). Knowledge, Attitude and Practice Among Midwives and Community Nurses on Cervical Cancer in The State of Kedah in 1997. *Community Health Journal*, 12(1).

Mattila, M. L., Rautava, P., Sillanpaa, M.,&Paunio, P. (2000). Caries in five-year-old children associated with family-related factor. *Journal of Dental Research, 79*, 879–881.

Masood S. A plea for a worldwide volunteer cervical cancer education and awareness program. *Acta Cytol* 1999;43:539-42.

Maxwell CJ, Bancej CM, Snider J, et al (2001). Factors important in promoting cervical cancer screening among canadian women: findings from the 1996-97 national population health survey (NPHS). *Can J Public Hlth*, 92, 127-33.

Mc Gain K. A & Hayloc P. J. Women's cancer: how to prevent them, how to treat them, how to beat them. New York: Hunter house inc, 2003.

Michael C. W. (1999). The Papanicolaou Smear and the Obstetric Patient: A Simple Test with Great Benefits. *Diagnostic Cytopathology*, 21(1). 64 Ministry of Health Malaysia. Malaysia's Health Technical Report of the Director-General of Health, Malaysia; 1999.

Ministry of Health, M., *Annual Report 2006*. 2006, Ministry of Health, Malaysia
Noor, M. R. (2008, 11 20). Retrieve 10 15, 2011, from Obgynanrush.com: http://site.obgynanrush.com/clients/obgynanrush/Downloads/Cervical Cancer Prevention in Malaysia by Rushdan for OGSM web112020081 22411PM.pdf

Narimah A, Rugayah HB, Tahir A, Maimunah AH: Cervical cancer screening, National Health and Morbidity Survey 1996 Volume 19. *Kuala Lumpur: Public Health Institute, Ministry of Health, Malaysia 1999.*

Nguyen, T., McPhee, S., Nguyen, T., Lam, T., & Mock, J. (2000). Predictors of cervical pap smear screening awareness, intention, and receipt among Vietnamese-American women. *American Journal of Preventive Medicine, 23*, 207–214.
Oon, S. W., Shuib, R., Ali, S. H., Nik Hussain, N. H., Shaaban, J., & Mohd Yusoff, H. (2010). Knowledge and Attitude among Women and Men in Decision Making on Pap Smear Screening in Kelantan, Malaysia. *World Academy of Science, Engineering and Technology*,66: 1660-1667.

Oscarsson, M. G., Wilma, B. F., & Benzein, E. G. (2008). " I Do Not Need To... I Do Not Want To... I Do Not Give It Priority..."- Why Women

Choose Not To Attend Cervical Cancer Screening. *Health Expect*, 11(1): 26-34.

Othman, P.D. *Cancer of the cervix- From Bleak Past To Bright Future; A review, With an Emphasis On Cancer Of The Cervix in Malaysia.*MAKNA
Scambler, G. (2004). Health and illness behavior. In Scambler, G. (Ed.), *Sociology as applied to medicine* (pp. 37–48). London: Saunders
Social Statistics Bulletin, Malaysia 2005. Kuala Lumpur; Department of Statistics, Malaysia;2005.

Stoppler M. C. "Who Should Get the HPV Vaccine?" *Medicine Net.com.*, 4 May2010. Web. 16 May 2012.
http://www.medicinenet.com/script/main/art.asp?articlekey=78889
Suls, J. M., & Goodkin, F. (1994). Medical gossip and rumor: Their role in the lay referral system. InR. F.Goodman&B.Ben-Ze'ev (Eds.), *Good gossip* (pp. 85–99). Lawrence, Kansas: University of Kansas Press.

Tang, T., Solomon, L., Yeah, C., & Worden, J. (1999). The role of cultural variables in breast self-examination and cervical cancer screening behavior in young 65 Asian women living in the United States. *Journal of Behavioral Medicine, 22*, 419–436.

Udigwe, G. O. (2006). Knowledge, Attitude and Practice of Cervical Cancer Screening (Pap Smear) Among Female Nurses In Nnewi, South Eastern Nigeria. *Nigerian Journal of Clinical Practice*, 9(1): 40-43.

Urasa, M., & Darj, E. (2011). Knowledge of Cervical Cancer and Screening Practices of Nurses at a Regional Hospital in Tanzania. *African Health Sciences*, 11(1): 48-57.

Wang, P. D., & Lin, R. S. (1996). Sociodemographic Factors of Pap Smear Screening in Taiwan. *Public Health*, 110(2): 123-127.

Williams, J. J., Santoso, J.T., Ling, F. W., & Przepiorka, D. (2003). Pap Smear Noncompliance Among Female Obstetrics-Gynecology Residents. *Gynecologic Oncology*, 90(3): 597-600.

Wong, L. P., Wong, Y. L., Low, W. Y., Khoo, E. M., & Shuib, R. (2008). Cervical Cancer Screening Attitudes and Beliefs of Malaysian Women who have Never had a Pap Smear: A Qualitative Study. *International Journal of Behavioural Medicine*, 15: 289-292.

Yu, C. K., & Rymer, J. (1998). Women's Attitudes To and Awareness of Smear Testing and Cervical Cancer. *Br j Fam Plann*, 23 (4): 127-33.

"Pap Smear: Pertahanan Terbaik melawan Kanser Serviks." Kotex Official Site. Web. Oct 2011

http://www.kotex.com.my/body-and-you-kesihatan/vagina/kanser-PAP-smear.aspx66

APPENDICES

PRACTICE AND BARRIERS TOWARDS PAP SMEAR SCEERING TEST
FOR CERVICAL CANCER

Please tick (√) for the following questions:

PART A: BACKGROUND.

1.Age:_____years old

2. Race: ☐Malay   ☐Chinese   ☐Indian Others:_____

3. Education level (*please tick your highest education level*)

☐ Never in school   ☐Primary school

☐ Secondary Middle School (Form 1-3)   ☐High School(Form

☐ Tertiary Education (Diploma, Bachelor, Master)

4. Occupation:

☐ Working. Please state:_____

☐ Housewife

☐ Self-employed (Please state:_____)

☐ Retired (Please state the previous
occupation:_____)

5. Husband's/partner's occupation:

☐ Working. Please state:_____

☐ Unemployed

☐ Self-employed (Please state:_____)

☐ Retired (Please state previous occupation:_____)

6. Home/family montly income estimation. Please state: RM_____)

7. Marital status

☐ Single ☐ Married ☐ Divorced ☐ Widowed

8. Age at the time of first marriage:_____ years old. ☐ Not married yet

		Yes	No	Not married yet
9.Is your current husband/partner is your first partner?		Yes	No	Not married yet
10.	You current husband/partner is your _____(number) of partner.			Not married yet
11.	Number of pregnancy (Including misscarriage):_____			
12.	Not married yet / Never have pregnancy / Have you had menopause? Yes No			
13.	How long has to been menopause? _____	Not menopause		
14.	Age at the time of menopause _____years	Not menopause		

PART B: THE PRACTICE OF PAP SMEAR TEST

15. Do you know about Pap Smear sceening test? ☐ Yes ☐ No

16. From which sourse did you know about Pap smear screening test?

		YES	NO
a.	Doctor/Hospital/Clinic		
b.	Printed Media (Newspaper, magazine, books, flyyers, etc)		
c.	Electronic Media (Radio, television etc)		
d.	Family/Relatives/Friends		
e.	Workplace/Employer		
f.	Internet		
g.	Others*		

*If yes, please state:_____ .

17. Have you undergo Pap smear
screening test?   Yes   No ☐   ☐

18. For how many times you undergo the Pap smear screening test?
_____

☐ Never doing Pap smer screening test.

19. How frequent do you undergo the Pap smear screening test?

☐ First time   ☐ Once a year

☐ Once in 2 years   ☐ Once in 3 years

☐ Never doing Pap smer screening test   Others:_____

20. When is your first Pap smear screening test?

☐ After married

☐ After first sexual intercourse

☐ After delivery

☐ After menopaused
After experiencing bleeding./ discharge
Never doing Pap smer screening test
Others:_____

21. In which year did you went for Pap smear screening test?
Year:_____

☐ Never doing Pap smer screening test

22. When is your last Pap smear screening test? Year:_____

☐ Never doing Pap smer screening test

23. Why did you undergo the Pap smear screening test

		YES	NO
a.	For health purpose		
b.	For detection of cervical cancer		
c.	From doctor's advise		
d.	Family/ Relatives/Friends/Employer influence		
e.	There are symptoms of cervical cancer		
f.	Want to conceive		
g.	Examination before pregnant		
h.	Examination after delivery		
i.	Family history of cervical cancer		
j.	Death of the family/relatives/ friends caused by cervical cancer		
k.	Others reason*		

* If yes, please state: _____ .

24. Why you not undergo Pap smear screening test?

		YES	NO
a.	Don't know/ Never heard about PST		
b.	Think it is not important		
c.	Fear		
d.	Emberassment		
e.	Don't care		
f.	No female doctor		
g.	Expansive		
h.	Don't have time/ busy		
i.	No encouragement from Husband/ Family/ Friends		
j.	Againts your Religion/Culture/ Principe		
k.	Distant Hospital/ Clinic		
l.	Painful		
m.	Pap smear makes me worry		

n.	Virginity will be taken away		
o.	Don't know where to get the Pap smear test		
p.	Others*		

*If yes, please state: _____ .

25. If you never have the test, have you ever think to

undergo Pap semar screening test? ☐ Yes ☐ No ☐
Already did it.

26. If you never have the Pap smear test, when is your planning of having a Pap smear screening test?

☐ A soon as possible   ☐ After recover/finish treatment   ☐ From d

☐ Not in the mind yet   ☐ Already did the Pap smear test   ☐ Never

PART C: THE KNOWLEDGE AND PERCEPTION TOWARDS PAP SEMAR SCREENING TEST.

27. What is the purpose of Pap Smear screening test?

☐ Detection of Cervical cancer   ☐ Dectection of sexual transmitted

☐ Detection of AIDS/HIV   ☐ Don't know

28. How often should Pap Smear screening test been done?

☐ One a year   ☐ Once in 1-3 years   ☐ Once in 5 years

73

☐ Once in a life time ☐ Don't know

29. In your opinion, which group of women that should undergo Pap Smear screening test?

		YES	NO
a.	Married		
b.	Not married		
c.	Have the family history of cervical cancer		
d.	Had menopause		
e.	Not yet menopause		
f.	Have the symptoms of cervical cancer		
g.	Want to conceive		
h.	Before delivery		
i.	After delivery		

30. Will you encourage women to undergo Pap Smear screening test?

☐ Yes   ☐ No   ☐ Don't know

31. Can women be forced to undergo the Pap Smear screening test?

☐ Yes   ☐ No   ☐ Don't know

32. Do you know that cervical cancer is caused by viral infection?

☐ Yes   ☐ No

33. Do you know that this infection is caused by sexual intercourse?

☐ Yes   ☐ No

THANK YOU

ABOUT THE AUTHOR

Redhwan Ahmed Al-Naggar obtained his PhD in community Medicine specialized in Epidemiology from the National University of Malaysia. Then he has obtained cancer prevention and control fellow from USA. He is working in Population Health and Preventive Medicine, Faculty of Medicine, Universiti Teknologi MARA (UiTM), Malaysia. He has published more than 156 original articles in refereed journals in more than a dozen journals, three books and produced more than 20 conference papers including international and national conferences. He is currently the Chief-editor of international Medical journals. Academic editor for PLOS, SCIENCEDOMAIN international, British Journal of Education, Society & Behavioural Science and others. Editorial board member for OMICS Group eBooks, Journal Community Medicine and Health Education, Journal of Pharmacy and Nutrition Sciences, Journal of Solid Tumors, Lifescience Global and others. Reviewer of local journals and international impact factor journal such as Asia Pacific journal of public Health, Journal of Peace, Gender and Development studies, Malaysian Journal of Medical Science, BMC Public Health, PLOS one, Vaccine Journal, BMC Research Notes, Journal of Solid Tumors, British Journal of Education, Society & Behavioural Science, BMC Women's Health, Medical Journal of Malaysia and others. In 2010 he was the winner of the best research Award in the Management and Science university, Malaysia which gives to the scientist who have mad outstanding contribution to the field of quantitative and qualitative research. Beside that supervise master and PhD students in community medicine field.